To all the midwives
supporting wa
unit

# WATER BIRTH

stories to inspire and inform

CW00421278

With love and best

wishes for the

future!

Sheena Byrom

2015

Published by Lonely Scribe
www.lonelyscribe.co.uk

First published 2014

Cover design and typesetting
copyright © 2014 Armadillo Design Ltd

ISBN: 978-1-905179-13-8

Front cover photograph © Rebecca Caroline,
birth photographer
**www.bambinoart.co.uk**

Back cover artwork © Helen Sargeant
**www.helensargeant.co.uk**

# WATER BIRTH

stories to inspire and inform

Edited by Milli Hill

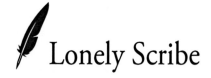

Lonely Scribe

*For my dad*

*who made me fall in love with words*

*and*

*Bess, Ursula and Albie*

*who made me fall in love with birth*

# Contents

# About the editor

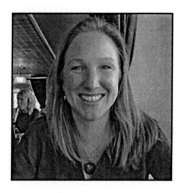

Milli Hill is a dramatherapist, trainee doula, writer and editor and the mother of three children, two born at home in water. She is the founder of the Positive Birth Movement, a network of free discussion groups set up to share support and information about birth, and she writes a weekly column about birth issues for *Best* magazine. Milli is also a contributor to *The Roar Behind The Silence*, a book that campaigns for improvements in maternity care.

# Acknowledgements

I would like to thank all of the people whose stories appear in this book, and the many more I was unable to include. Each and every story, whether it made the book or not, was inspirational and informative and I am very grateful to all of you for sharing the details of such an intimate and special moment of your lives.

I'd also like to thank the lovely and patient Susan Last for asking me to edit this book, and my mum Pauline Hill for helping me to proofread the stories.

Special thanks must go to the man I love, George Litchfield, who is the most amazing supporter – whether I am giving birth to a book or a baby, he somehow manages to stay calm, believe in me and let me do my thing.

# Introduction

Conversations about birth rarely take place in our culture without mention of pain. Pregnant women are often asked, 'What are you going to do about pain relief?' Antenatal classes talk women through the options: gas and air, pethidine, epidural. Television dramas – both real and fictional – offer images of women in distress, 'begging for drugs'. This focus is interesting, and unique to birth. Others who are about to undertake a great feat of human endurance and achievement – marathon runners, mountain explorers, Olympic athletes and so on – are not asked to focus so persistently on the question of what they might do in the moments they feel they cannot cope or continue. But for pregnant women, this is considered a key question.

Water birth is far from exempt from this cultural habit. Indeed, it is often described as – and marketed as – a 'form of pain relief'. The experience of pain is, of course, hard to quantify or measure; nevertheless researchers seem to agree that getting into a birth pool can help with the discomfort of labour – a 2009 Cochrane review, for example, found that water birth significantly reduced the need for epidural anaesthesia. Perhaps more powerful than such studies is the anecdotal evidence – with which this book is filled – that getting into a pool of warm water makes labour easier:

*'As the water lapped against my body and the warmth penetrated my skin I felt all the tension melt away and with it all pain.'*

*'At no point at all was I tempted to ask for medical pain relief.'*

*'As soon as the water touched my skin I felt instant relief.'*

*'Yes, it hurts, but it's manageable. The water – somehow taking away the rawness.'*

Pain is complicated. One woman may describe birth as blissful while the next proclaims it unbearable, and we have no real way of measuring accurately whether there is any tangible difference between the two. In 1942, Dr Grantly Dick-Read wrote his groundbreaking book, *Childbirth Without Fear*, in which he described the Fear-Tension-Pain cycle. Put simply, Dick-Read suggests that it is fear in labour that causes us to experience true pain – which in turn makes us more afraid – and the pain worsens. Labouring women can become trapped in this vicious circle, from which the only escape is pain-relieving drugs.

Water birth is a form of pain relief… it seems this much is true; however, reading the stories in this book, and the countless others I have been sent but have not had space for, I can't help but feel that this is a bit reductionist – placing the birth pool in the category of 'equipment', 'tool' or 'pain relief option', when clearly it transcends this and is much, much more. To talk about birth pools as pain relief is to keep the body and mind separate, when, as Dick-Read knew – and all birthing women know – they are not. Giving birth is not just a physical experience; like running a marathon, it is also mental and emotional, and fear or doubt can hold us back just as courage can urge us onwards.

Stepping into a birth pool makes a series of statements. It says, 'I want to do this myself, I want to do this without intervention, I want to be in tune with my body and with nature'. It also says, 'If you want to join me in my experience, you are going to have to get wet'. Birth pools create a protected distance between the labouring woman and the rest of the world, and the moment her body enters the water she reclaims a great deal of the power that has been taken by the over-medicalisation of birth in the past fifty or so years.

Interestingly, there seem to be attempts to take back this power from the woman in the birth pool. Protocols in hospital water birth often dictate that a woman may only get in the water once she has reached a certain dilation, because, she is told, the water may slow her labour. But messages are mixed. The same woman wishing for a conventional hospital birth might be told to stay home and take a bath in early labour, whilst others are told not to get into their birth pool at home until the midwives arrive, in case the effect of the water is to 'speed them up'.

Policy and protocol varies, but access to the pool itself remains a problem, with women reporting being told they are 'not allowed' a birth in water for a variety of reasons, and with those who are assessed to be suitable often finding that, on the day of their labour, the pool is off-limits for practical reasons such as staff shortages or plumbing issues. Still others find they are told to get out of the water for vaginal exams or due to concerns over time or progress.

Giving birth in water is effectively a counter-cultural choice, and as such, is liable to make some uncomfortable and be met with opposition and obstacles. Whether it's your husband who thinks it's 'all a bit wacky', a cynical aunt who questions safety, or your healthcare provider who feels you are not a suitable candidate, you might have to fight to have your water birth, or even to get in and out of the water when you choose.

Fortunately you will find you are supported by a growing movement embodied in organisations such as Birthrights, which supports a woman's legal and human right to birth where and how she wishes. With the choice to birth in water, as with all other choices you make about your pregnancy, labour and birth, you have the right to do your own homework, be fully informed by the professionals caring for you, and then to have the final say in what happens to you, your body and your baby.

Stepping over the threshold of the birth pool provides a retreat from all such concerns. This brings the relief that many describe; not just 'pain relief', but relief that you are in your safe place, your sanctuary. Many of the stories in this book are of so-called 'healing births': women who have had traumatic experiences with their first babies, and who have chosen the birth pool as a place to rediscover the power that they feel was taken out of their hands the first time around.

It's a shame it has to be this way, but in our current birth environment, women need to work hard to find a place they feel safe, dignified and protected when they have their babies. Privacy – so essential in all mammalian birth – is also a major issue: contrast the often starkly lit hospital delivery room, with what has been described as the 'big dark skirts' of the birth pool.

It's no coincidence, I believe, that the rise in water birth directly mirrors the rise in birth interventions in the past twenty or thirty years. As normal birth rates have fallen, more and more women have chosen to birth in water (see the graph opposite).

Of course, superficially this is about privacy, alternative pain relief, and the desire for the best chance of normality. But, if we look deeper, I think that women's desire to give birth in water is also representing something at a symbolic level.

Water is an archetypal symbol of the highest order: all life once emerged from it, and throughout time and across cultures, water has represented the life source, healing, and the sacred feminine. Add to this the shape of the birth pool, and you have a circle – a symbol of the goddess, the feminine, and wholeness or completeness. A circle full of water.

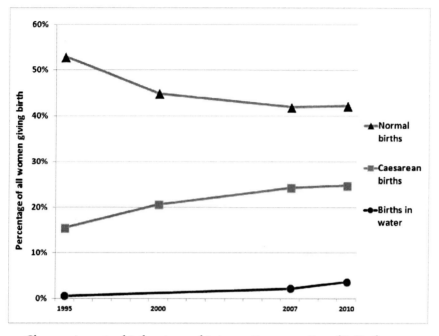

*Changes in water birth rates and interventions over time (© Birth-ChoiceUK, 2013).* [1]

Against a backdrop of what has been called the 'medicalisation' or even the 'masculinisation' of childbirth, women step into this circle full of water to reclaim their power. A circle full of water, a feminine place of sanctuary, from which, after a true heroine's journey full of doubt and challenges, new life triumphantly emerges. In this watery and magical ring, a child is born, and so is a mother.

Of course, if all of this sounds a bit far-fetched, you are welcome to refer to your birth pool as a form of pain relief, for, as you will read in this book, your reasons for choosing water birth will not alter its effect. And it could well be that you will not fully understand the meaning of water birth to you personally until you step over that threshold into your watery nest.

For now, dip into the pages of this book or take time to completely immerse yourself in the wonderful and varied stories here, for the very best way to learn about birth is to hear positive stories from other women who have been there and come back eager to tell you their oxytocin-rich story.

And so… let them begin… starting with my own…

NB. *Terms marked with an asterisk (\*) are explained in the Gloassary at the end of the book.*

---

1. Graph prepared using data from the following sources:

Caesarean birth rates: Health and Social Care Information Centre (2012) NHS Maternity Statistics, England 2011-12.

Water birth rates: 1995: Gilbert and Tookey (1999); 2007: Health Care Commission Maternity Services Review 2007; 2010: Care Quality Commission Maternity Services Survey 2010

Normal birth rates: Derived from Health and Social Care Information Centre Hospital Episode Statistics (HES) records using the Maternity Care Working Party consensus definition of normal birth (2007)

**References:**

Gilbert, R.E., Tookey, P.A. (1999) 'Perinatal mortality and morbidity among babies delivered in water: surveillance study and postal survey'. BMJ 1999; 319: 483–7

Maternity Care Working Party (2007). *Making normal birth a reality. Consensus statement from the Maternity Care Working Party: our shared views about the need to recognise, facilitate and audit normal birth.* National Childbirth Trust; Royal College of Midwives; Royal College of Obstetricians and Gynaecologists.

# Milli Hill

I first heard about water birth in my first pregnancy, during which I planned to deliver at home. I must admit, I was entirely skeptical – it sounded like a bit of a 'fad' to me, and my feeling was that if womankind had been managing to have babies perfectly well for millennia without a hundred and fifty quids worth of inflatable rubber involved, then I could do the same.

Added to this was the advice, which I heard consistently: if you like having a bath for period pain, then you will like water birth. I didn't really get period pain, but on the rare occasions I did, I was more of a hot-water bottle under the duvet kind of girl. I decided against a pool. Besides, it would barely fit in our tiny living room, and I feared that even if it did, my birthing bottom might be rather too near the letterbox for my liking.

In the end, the thought and planning I put into my home birth was largely wasted, as I fell into the 'Induction Trap', coming under pressure from just a few days 'overdue', a pressure so intense that I think it's unlikely I could ever have gone into labour. Eventually, tearful, uncomfortable and desperate to do the right thing, I agreed to be induced in hospital, and my beautiful daughter Bess was born 18 days after her estimated due date.

My labour was intense, but I chose not to have 'pain relief', and instead chanted a lot and spent some time in the large hospital bath. Everything seemed to be going well, until, towards the end, it was decided that things were taking too much time. A man in a suit was called, and after an examination that I found incredibly traumatic, he declared she was 'OP', or 'back to back'. My labour ended with feet in stirrups, an episiotomy*, and a brief forceps delivery. Looking at the notes now it is clear that the birth was pretty imminent when this happened, and with the beauty of hindsight, I do rather wish that those in charge of my care had put their efforts into helping me into new positions and feeding me a bit of banana, rather than resorting to what always seems to me a rather medieval solution to the 'problem'.

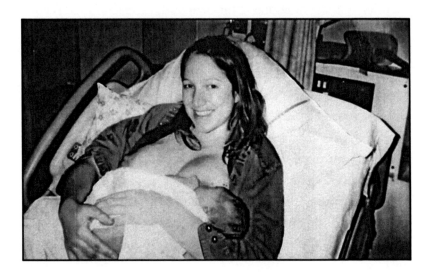

In spite of the trauma, I bonded and breastfed well with my daughter, although I think I was more than usually anxious in my first few months of motherhood, due in part to my feeling 'shell-shocked' from the somewhat rough and forced nature of her beginning. But as time went by, I did begin to dwell a little less on what had happened, and it wasn't until I became pregnant again two years later that my thoughts turned back to birth. Weirdly, although I was a mother already, there were two things I felt I had never done – gone into labour or pushed a baby out. So I began to worry – was I actually capable of either of these?

I decided to have a rethink about water birth. By this time quite a few friends had given birth in pools and they all raved about it. Added to this, we had moved to a larger house and fitting the pool in was more practically possible, so I planned a home water birth with NHS midwives. However, quite a long way into my pregnancy my local midwifery system changed from community midwifery to a 'bank' system, and I discovered that I might be attended by a midwife with no experience of home or water birth.

Since I had such doubts in my own capabilities I wanted to be sure that my midwife, at least, knew what she was doing. We took the decision to hire an Independent Midwife*, which turned out to be one of the best choices we ever made. The one-to-one care they offered meant that they had time to help me process my first daughter's birth, and prepare myself for a different experience, that they assured me would be 'healing'. Their attitude to birth was filled with confidence, and they filled me with confidence too. They also didn't bat an eyelid when I went nearly two weeks past my 'due date', and, as I had requested, didn't even offer a sweep.

However, that time of waiting was hard for me. I felt huge, and cumbersome, and worst of all, riddled with doubt. I feared that there was something wrong with me, a 'switch missing', that meant I would never go into labour spontaneously, and as each day passed I became more and more despondent. In spite of this, I did manage to avoid all of the 'natural induction methods' that I had become caught up in last time, and focused instead on what I felt might be psychological blocks that were holding me back. I developed a mantra, 'I am ready to let go', which seemed to make a good antidote to the anxious control freak aspect of my personality. I bounced on my birth ball, letting the baby's head knock on the door of my cervix, and repeated it, over and over.

In the early hours of the morning on 27 May, I was woken by some very strong sensations. I had been asleep on a mattress on the floor with my daughter Bess, so crept away to my partner George and woke him up. Could something be happening? We went downstairs together in the dark and chatted and waited for more and wondered what to do. The tightenings were intermittent, and eventually we put in a quick call to our midwife Chrissy, who advised we went back to bed.

The next morning, there still seemed to be some activity, but it was patchy. Some sensations felt powerful, others like Braxton Hicks, and there was no real pattern. As we had an immersion tank hot water system, we decided to start filling the pool just in case, as we had already had a trial run and it had taken several hours.

By late morning there was still not much happening, and of course I remained full of doubt in my body and convinced it would all just fizzle out, as had happened to me a few times in my first pregnancy. I felt extremely hungry, and had a huge and sudden craving for a fry up that absolutely had to include sausages. My lovely partner obeyed with a trip to the butcher, and after my desire for 'pig and egg' had been sated, I took myself off to bed for a nap.

When I woke I felt different. Somehow I just knew this was it. I went to the bathroom and tied my hair back. I can remember thinking – rather vainly – that I had better make an effort to make it look nice as I would be having my picture taken later holding my baby!

While I had been asleep George had tidied up the house and put a vase of fresh lilac on the kitchen table, which I found very touching. He also started making vegetable soup – it all sounds idyllic, right?! As he finely diced courgettes I found myself having a really serious, I-Mean-Business contraction, kneeling on the floor of the living room, leaning on an armchair, with the two-year-old climbing on my back and the dog, who never likes to be left out, placing a slobbery ball in front of my face. I'm afraid I shattered the moment by yelling, 'Stop making ****ing soup and get rid of this ****ing dog!' at the top of my lungs.

Suddenly we both realised that something really was happening. The dog was banished to our neighbours. George's sister Caroline came to take care of Bess. The midwives were called. I lit some candles and put on some music. By myself in the living room, this felt like a good moment! I was actually in labour! I didn't have a missing switch after all! And all this time the pool was sitting ready, kept warm by a cover – but I didn't want to get in until the midwives arrived. They had a long distance to come, over an hour's drive, and I was worried that the pool could speed up my labour and mean I delivered before they got to me. Whether or not this would have been the case, we will never know – but I was happy to err on the side of caution as I desperately wanted their presence.

Time passed, and they did not arrive. My labour intensified. They rang to say they were stuck in traffic. I kept trying to chant, as I had in my first labour, but somehow it just didn't work this time, and felt like wasted energy. By just before 6pm I was on the sofa, struggling to find comfort and feeling really panicked by the absence of midwives. George was with me, and I started to cry. Where were they?! And then, suddenly, they both came through the back door, their arms outstretched in reassurance and comfort. They both put their hands on me, they were warm, and motherly, and I suddenly felt that everything would be alright.

After briefly checking me and the baby (but no VE's*, at my request), they suggested I get in the pool. That was by far and away one of the most wonderful moments of my life. I felt as if so much pain and anxiety was just washed away by the water, like being really muddy, and then getting clean again. I realised, in that moment, that water birth is not just a fad, and it's not really about 'pain relief', like having a bath when you've got your period. It's far deeper than that – it's a sanctuary, a place of safety, a watery nest where no one can reach you and where power is rightfully restored.

It's funny, but although my time in the pool was only an hour and three quarters, it's really my only true memory of labour. For those couple of hours, I felt as if all my perceptions were heightened, like moving from black and white to technicolour. Suddenly I was able to flip my enormously pregnant body into whatever position felt best with ease and grace. My midwife Chrissy knelt by the pool and helped me through each contraction, guiding me in a low, gentle tone, which was just what I needed. I was really in my element.

The room seemed to be full of lightness and love. At one point I asked Chrissy if she had dropped a torch in the pool, as it seemed suddenly illuminated in an otherwise fairly dark room. She hadn't, but a chink of light from the spring evening sunshine had come through the curtains, striking the pool at just the right angle and making it glow an ethereal blue. We all marvelled at this for some time, and even took photos. It felt like a nod of approval from Mother Nature herself.

Shortly after that my daughter returned from a walk with her Aunty, and brought me a bunch of hedgerow flowers – cow parsley, buttercups and red campion. I had been worried about what to do with her during a home birth, but it couldn't have been lovelier than to have her around, dipping in and out of the birth room and reminding me of what I was working towards. I felt huge waves of love for her, for my partner, and for everyone present!

Emotions ran high and deep. In the midst of all the love I was working through my fears and trauma from my previous birth.

I began to feel that the 'pushing stage' was imminent, and this frightened me. I was scared I couldn't do it, and scared that I could! What would it feel like? It seemed an impossible feat. I really cried and the midwives and George gave me much-needed reassurance.

My waters did not break until right near the end, in the pool. I also had a wee once or twice in the water. I highly recommend this to all water birthers – it feels a bit odd but it is well diluted by the pool and it certainly beats what must be an agonising trip to the loo. To give birth we really need to let go of concerns about what others think of us or what we should or shouldn't do. Weeing in the pool was quite liberating in this respect for me.

And then the 'pushing stage' began, the ultimate in letting go. I was not a quiet birther who breathed her baby down into the world in tranquility. I roared. I gripped hard onto George's arms, and he gripped mine, and I knelt and I pulled back on his arms with all my might and I roared. I felt extremely powerful, and extremely determined. If I could have talked I might have shouted, 'You are not going to get me this time you ****ers!'. I felt I was taking on the demons of my trauma in that moment, and reclaiming the strength they had – briefly – taken from me.

Chrissy asked me if I wanted to catch the baby. To me this seemed like a ridiculous suggestion. 'Nooooo! I'M...TOO... BUSY!!!' I remember saying, so she gently passed her up to me through the water. We looked to see what we had – a girl. I held her, repeating incredulously, 'I did it! I did it!'. I couldn't believe that it was over and that I had done it all myself. I felt elated.

I was aware that the midwives were repeating to me to rub my baby, and to talk to her, as if they were perhaps a little concerned, but I knew that she was fine. She soon began to make more visible signs of breathing, and suddenly my other daughter was in the room, and everyone was marvelling in excitement at the new person present. George ripped off his clothes and jumped in the water to be closer to us, and Bess was helped out of her pyjamas so she could do the same. It was an incredible moment – the four of us – a woman empowered and a family made new, in the very healing waters.

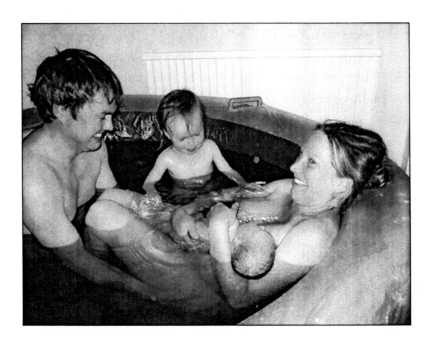

# Michel Odent

*Michel Odent, MD, is a pioneer and as such has been influencing childbirth for several decades, perhaps most notably by introducing the concept of birth pools to the world. He founded the Primal Health Research Centre and is currently particularly interested in how the rapidly changing way that babies are born might affect the evolution of our species. He is the author of over fifty scientific papers, including the first article in the medical literature about initiating breastfeeding during the hour following birth. His thirteen books include* Water and Sexuality, Birth Reborn, *and, most recently,* Childbirth and the Future of Homo Sapiens.*

*Here Michel shares two anecdotes about birth in water. In the first, his belief in the powerful and symbolic influence of water on the birthing woman shines through the simplicity of the story. In the second, his humour cuts through the often many and various concerns about water birth safety, normalising the natural and involuntary process of birth.*

## First anecdote

Michelle has rented a birthing pool for the home birth of her first baby. At the last minute, when the labour is well established, it appears that a device connecting the pool to the tap is missing. It seems impossible to fill up the pool the normal way. Michelle's husband is condemned to overcome this technical difficulty by using a saucepan. At the very time when the bath is finally available, the baby is born.

The grandmother of Michelle had also given birth at home. During several hours her husband had been boiling water.

Two variants of the same story: busy husbands and noise of water in the birthing places.

## Second anecdote

At the very end of a conference, a last-minute question.

**Q:** What are the contraindications for the use of birthing pools?

**A:** One contraindication: easy and fast birth on the dry land.

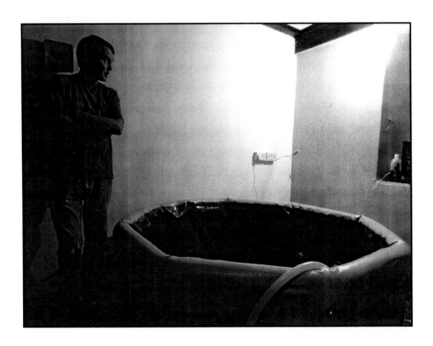

# Lisa Hassan Scott

*Having given birth to her first child in her local hospital, Lisa Hassan Scott chose a birthing pool at home for her next two deliveries. Lisa is a yoga teacher and freelance writer. She lives in Wales with her husband and three children and writes a successful blog about parenting and the mind.*

## Lisa's Story

From this distance, my water births seem so run-of-the-mill. What to say about experiences that have, to me, come to feel so ordinary and usual? I have to remind myself that water birth is truly an extraordinary thing; indeed, for many people who see birth interventions as normal, even a natural birth is unusual.

I have three children and gave birth to two of them in water. My first was an intense, beautiful, natural birth in my local hospital. I tore badly and lost a lot of blood. Weak and thirsty afterwards, the midwives sent my husband home and me to a cramped ward full of beleaguered-looking mothers and their babies in little plastic boxes. I was bewildered and unsure; the midwives were busy and short-tempered. Ultimately, my baby and I were alone.

I was the only mother on the ward who wanted to breast-feed. In the night, as my daughter and I worked to latch her on, I listened to other babies screaming as they waited for their bottles. They woke me even when my own baby was sleeping. There was no privacy: every time I drew the curtain around my bed, a midwife would click it open in annoyance.

When I became pregnant again, I knew I wanted different post-natal experiences. I chose a home birth.

A close friend had used a birthing pool for one of her births, and I fell in love with the idea. A swimmer from a very young age, I have a natural affinity with the water. But more than this, I wanted to be in charge of my own space. I am fiercely independent (some might say I'm stubborn), and although I wanted support in labour, I knew that ultimately only I could birth this baby. A birthing pool sounded to me like a wonderful way to have my own personal space: no one else could come into it unless I consented.

To say that I was unusual is an understatement. At the time, in my area, only one NHS midwife had experience of water birth and it was the luck of the draw whether she was available when you went into labour. My local midwifery team had no under-water dopplers: I'd have to rise up out of the water whenever they wanted to check the baby's heartbeat. They'd started to develop guidelines, and I seemed to be their guinea pig. At each appointment, a different midwife would attend and tell me something different. Many times there was confrontation.

It was hard to stand my ground. After those appointments I cried tears of frustration. I knew what I wanted and had faith in myself to birth my baby, but my team of health professionals seemed determined to own my birth.

In the end, I owned my baby's birth. After only a few hours of labour, I laughed joyfully when the midwife arrived and confirmed that my cervix was 8cm dilated. We'd drawn the curtains in our conservatory, where we'd set up the pool. Keith had the temperature just right. I can vividly remember the 'Ahhhhhhh' as the water touched my skin. My pool was a familiar place because I'd spent many evenings in it meditating, chanting, listening to music and floating. As I rode through the contractions, I returned to that trance-like state I'd practised on so many evenings. I held my husband's hand and went through transition: the most intensely frightening experience I've ever had before or since. One of the midwives murmured, 'You'll be pushing soon'. And I knew that my body wasn't going to tear in half, as I'd thought. No, I would be giving birth right here, in a few moments. Several pushes later, my daughter emerged. She lay at the bottom of the pool and I gazed at her. The midwife reached in and grabbed her, handed her to me and an ebullient cry rose from my chest to meet my daughter's tiny whimper. Hers was the sound of a gently-born baby. Mine was the sound of a woman who had found her power.

When I became pregnant again, this time in a different house, we put the birthing pool in the centre of our sitting room. The girls and I played in it, relaxed in it, and after they went to bed I meditated upon a photograph of a lotus flower that I'd pinned to the wall at eye level. I didn't bother worrying about what the midwives said and, by this time, the health authority had finally woken up to the benefits of water birth, so they were trying to learn more about it. Because my previous experience was well-known for being so unique, the midwives knew I had more experience than them in this area.

After many false starts, I went into labour. I walked my eldest the three miles to and from school, took my youngest to the park and counted minutes between contractions. Finally I decided to go home and begin making preparations for the arrival of our third child. Keith came home from work, we collected my daughter from school and we went home to make a family dinner. It was just a normal day, but every so often I stopped to concentrate fully on my body as a contraction drew me away from the reality of family life toward the internal processes happening for my baby and me. A friend agreed to look after the girls. Keith and I lit the log-burner, heated the pool and had a lovely time together. This baby was back-to-back, so my labour was long, slow and intense. I often had to slow things down by going onto all fours, putting my head to the floor and sticking my bottom into the air.

I became tired, drank smoothies for energy and ate dry cereal.

Eventually, I felt a little like I wanted to push. I asked Keith to call the midwives, and by the time they arrived I was stripping off to get in the pool. I knew that one of the signs of the onset of the second stage of labour was a loss of inhibition, so I knew I would be meeting my baby soon.

I felt the same sense of total relaxation and comfort when I stepped into the pool. Two midwives and a student midwife stood a short distance away. The midwives chatted quietly and left me to my own devices; I was grateful that the pool was my sanctuary. Keith crouched beside me, just outside the pool. There was a lull in contractions, and then I felt a strong urge to push.

I put my hand to my perineum when I felt the baby's head crown; there was no pain, just a numbness. I felt myself opening. I told myself, 'One more push and you will meet your new child'. That thought filled me with such elation that I pushed my baby's head halfway out, then completely out on the next push. I laughed, looked down and saw a small black head. I touched that soft warm head, pushed again and lifted my baby's slippery little body to my chest. Lying there, that purple blue wrinkled skin enveloped an old soul. I touched my baby all over, and with surprise felt something between those little skinny legs. 'It's a boy! We have a boy!' I said. It was a moment I will forever treasure in the quiet spaces of my heart.

The next day, my midwife visited and showed me my birth notes. 'Here, where it says "Who delivered the baby?" I wanted to write "MOTHER" but the form only gives you the option of "midwife" or "doctor",' she said. 'I put "midwife", but it wasn't me, it was you.' I looked down at my son sleeping on my bare chest, as serene as he was the moment after he was born, and I knew that I'd birthed him. It was me, on my terms, in my space. Even now, I can feel the power and taste the satisfaction.

# Natasha Hodge

*Natasha Hodge had planned to have her first baby at home but this ended in
a transfer to hospital. Determined not to experience a hospital birth again, she
went on to deliver her second child at home in water. When Natasha found
out she was having twins she knew she would face opposition to have them at
home, but with support from family, friends and both NHS and Independent
Midwives, she went on to have one of the few planned home water twin births
in the UK. Natasha lives in Plymouth with her partner and four children.*

## Natasha's Story

During the week building up to the birth, I was woken up by
lower backache and frequent trips to the toilet. I was still feeling
sick most evenings, which wasn't fun either, and along with
pelvic pain and three-point-turns to get out of bed, I was feeling
pretty fed up.

Having already been told at 35 weeks that I was four centimetres, I was thinking every night that this was going to be it.
But of course it wasn't, and every morning I'd wake shattered
and wondering when it was all going to kick off, but also hoping
that they would stay put until the following week when I would
turn 37 weeks.

The following Monday at 37 weeks at two in the morning the
backache was stronger. I had several trips to the loo and I started
losing bloody show. I had been losing my plug for weeks but
this was the first sign that labour was not too far away. I went
back to bed feeling like this could be it, but fell asleep and in the
morning it had all stopped. I felt odd… it was the quiet before
the storm!

My midwife Cheryl rang and said she would come and see me and she did my blood pressure and wee and everything was fine. She wrote on my notes that things were probably not far off and I felt quite teary when she left – I just couldn't put my finger on why I felt so weird.

I really didn't feel labour was going to come but still I informed Nicky, the Independent Midwife* whom I had invited to the birth. Nicky had never been to a twin home birth and had been a great support to me in getting my home birth through the NHS. I told her it was likely to happen that week, and while still feeling odd I also felt very tired, so had an early night.

*  *  *  *  *

It's around 5am and I get woken up by a huge urge to go to the toilet. I sit there in disbelief that I have slept from 9pm until 5am without a trip to the loo – maybe the urgency was because of that? I have quite intense lower backache, but still in denial I just put it down to Twin 1 being posterior, but then I feel a surge in my lower back that doesn't go away… and then I have lots more bloody show… still sat there thinking am I?… and then another intense surge… YES I AM!

I run downstairs… well no – I waddle – who am I kidding! I tell my husband Paul I'm in labour and by this point the backache feels constant and quite intense but still totally manageable. I get him to ring maternity while I let Nicky know what's happening so that she can make her way once the midwives have come.

At around 6am Cheryl arrives. We make our way upstairs to check on my blood pressure and the babies. I have a few 'back contractions' and she suggests having a check of my dilation.

I lie back on my bed and I then get informed I'm at 9cm…

9cm!!! Wow – I got to 9cm without much discomfort?! Cheryl tells me it's unlikely I'll make it into the pool. I go downstairs to inform Paul while in total shock and urge him to get going with the pool quick!

Then the Supervisor of Midwives (SOM) turns up and around ten minutes later a hospital midwife. I feel in a fluster but the SOM and hospital midwife take over and sort out my daughter Olivia's lunch and hair for school (ha ha! NOT on the job description but so thankful they did that!)

From here everything is quite hazy…

So here I am labouring away, and at some point I remember Nicky turning up and someone else… I think. It was around 8am now and Olivia had gone to school. Charlotte my smallest was in her element being fussed over, while I'm over a chair still with back pain and really wanting to get in that pool!

The contractions, which until now had been in my back, had started to move round to the front. They were coming and going – short, and without a real pattern – but I trusted they were doing what was needed.

Suddenly, the pool was ready! I got in and my goodness it felt GOOD! I had a few more contractions in there.

I looked up at the clock – it was nearly 9. I was waiting for my Mum to turn up and deep down didn't want anything to happen without her there. I think around ten minutes later I saw her come through the front room door and I knew then I wasn't far off from having my babies.

The contractions stalled and Cheryl suggested I stood up. My waters still hadn't gone, and I felt that it was likely she was still trying to turn. I got out of the pool and felt like I needed a wee so I went upstairs – it felt like she was going to fall out! I managed to do a little wee and came back down after a contraction on the loo.

Sue suggested I get on the ball and do some pelvic rolls; the contractions returned both back and front and were really intense now. I was still able to breathe through them and was wishing my waters would just go… they didn't, and feeling frustrated I got off the ball and tried squatting. This was really uncomfortable so I gave up with that, and Cheryl said she would like to try some reflexology. While Cheryl did this I had some very intense contractions, but still no water breaking. Cheryl said it might be an idea to break my waters, as although the contractions were there they were still infrequent or short and I think she could see how fed up I was. I said I'd had enough and wanted to get back in the pool. Cheryl suggested breaking my waters first if I wanted and my head just screamed 'YES!'

She checked me first and said I was complete and little lady's head was 'right there' – bag bulging. She got everything ready, and after what seemed like forever I felt a gush! And it felt great! Instant relief!

The contractions changed and I felt like I had moved right on to the next stage. I got back in the pool and got in a hands and knees position and the contractions now felt like my back was being torn in two. I got Paul to put pressure on my back (he put his whole weight on me and it still didn't feel enough). I was feeling weepy now (ahhhh transition…) – fed up and so over it! I tried doing little pushes to see if it would help but it felt like they were doing nothing.

I moved round to sitting up to see if this would help, but it didn't and the contractions were very hard and intense so I moved back round to all fours and the urge to push started. I vaguely remember hearing that it might be good to stand up or get out of the pool as the contractions were spreading out again, but I didn't want to and just ignored what was being said. I felt really weepy and pathetic and just really fed up. I was pushing and getting Paul to push on my back but it felt like it was doing nothing; the pushing felt ineffective and the pushing on my back was really not cutting it either.

The pain was too intense now and the whole time I was just thinking 'I could really do with some gas and air and why am I not asking for it?!' I continued to debate this in my head whilst being very vocal about how I really didn't want to do this anymore. I also remember saying to myself, 'Why am I not having this pain-free birth I've read about?! What did I do wrong?!! Orgasmic birth my ass!'

I moved back round as I wanted to birth little lady in a sitting position. I held onto the handles and asked Paul to hold onto my shoulders, but he was doing it wrong and I told him to get off! So my Mum stepped in and said she would. The pushing and contractions felt unbearable and so hard, I was shouting at this point and feeling so so fed up. The contractions now felt constant and there was no relief even when pushing. Finally, I heard that they could see her, but after I stopped pushing I could feel her move back up. I felt like I was never going to get her out! Still pushing down I seemed to be getting closer but it was getting more and more intense – I couldn't do it anymore, I didn't want to be there anymore and I didn't want to push anymore.

I heard Cheryl tell me to breathe through them and stop pushing (I guess she was near crowning) but Paul was saying push and I vaguely remember telling him to f***ing shut up (whoops!).

Then I could feel it, her head was coming and wow was it intense, I just wanted her out! And finally her head was! RELIEF! I put my hands down and touched her soft little head and I could feel her wriggling and turning. I had another contraction, and she was out. I got hold of her and pulled her up to my chest, she looked just like Charlotte… my heart melted!

This feeling was soon overtaken by very, very intense contractions and I asked for her cord to be cut. Paul took off his top for some skin-to-skin and Sue said she would like to hold little man in place to prevent him turning (now he had all that room!). At that point I didn't care as it was just so intense and I felt like I couldn't do it. I got on all fours and just pushed; there wasn't much of an urge but I wanted him out! There was no break at all between contractions and I felt like my body was going to give up. I suddenly felt his head and felt the burning as he crowned, he wriggled and I heard that the caul was still intact! He wriggled some more and as I pushed again he shot out and it broke.

Cheryl passed him through my legs and as I grabbed him I was overcome with every emotion I could have possibly felt! I brought him up and couldn't believe how small he was and so perfect! Part of his sac was floating off his arm and I was totally in awe! After having three girls, I just couldn't get over seeing this little boy.

A little while after I felt really uncomfortable and felt the need to have his cord cut and get out of the pool.

I had to hold onto my stomach (it felt like everything was going to drop out) and my Mum helped me get out of the pool and over to the sofa. I sat down and was still getting contractions – the placentas were on their way.

Paul brought in the boxes we had for them as I had Lesley coming round after (from IPEN Placenta Network) to encapsulate the placentas and do me a smoothie. I gave a little push and out it came!

The placentas were fused and looked very healthy, the bleeding was quite minimal and I sat back on the sofa while everyone was sorting out bits around me. This is now quite a blur as I felt really drained by this point. The bleeding got a little heavier so

I consented to having syntometrine. A few minutes after this I started being sick and felt pretty awful.

Both then had a little feed while the other was being weighed. Megan came out at 5lb 7oz and Jack 4lb 11oz. Transitional care was mentioned but I said no and that I would try and see how things went. I felt deep down I was more than capable of keeping them warm and both had taken to the breast easily so I wasn't worried.

I was sick again and was feeling so crap. Cheryl suggested having a bath so I went up and sat on the toilet while waiting for it to fill. I got in and felt like my body melted, it was just what I needed. I asked Paul to put in a few drops of lavender and just relaxed for a little bit.

I let the bath drain before having a shower and washing my hair; my body felt empty and heavy and I needed to get into bed. I got out of the shower to find Cheryl had put some pads on the bed and I just got right in, it felt good to be there.

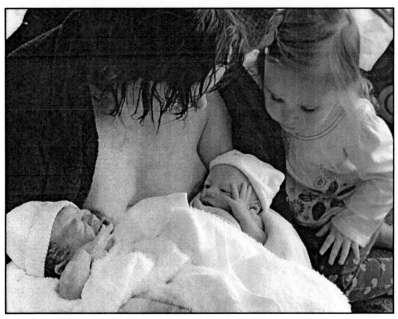

Paul brought Megan and Jack up and I had a cuddle with them, people started to leave and everything was being tidied up around me.

Some point after Cheryl did some more checks and then got her bits together to set off, and an hour later I heard Lesley arrive to make my placenta smoothie! She came up the stairs with such a lovely energy and I knew I was going to like this drink!

The smoothie had both Megan and Jack's placentas in it; I tried one sip and all I could taste was lovely fruit. Still in a daze (and overwhelmed) we had a little chat about the birth. It felt so right to have her be there and be a part of the birth experience.

Within the hour I felt so much better! The drink was amazing! I am so so glad that I had it. There was also another glass for the next day too so I knew I would have another pick-me-up and boy would I need it!

That night I had no sleep. Megan fed and fed and I found it hard to try and get Jack to feed. He was very mucousy but I wasn't going to give up! Finally at 6am when it finally clicked to try skin-to-skin he had a great long feed! I felt so relieved. Both are now doing very very well and both feed like pros! I'm glad I followed my instincts.

# Emily Hunter

*Emily Hunter chose a birth program that provided an integrated model of care; midwives, doctors and doulas working together. She gave birth to Jonah in water and describes the labour as hard work — not painful — but exhilarating and empowering. Emily is a freelance writer and researcher and lives in Vancouver, British Columbia, Canada with her husband, David, and young son, Jonah.*

## Water birth poem for Jonah

Poppy seed spark, you flickered unsteadily
in the watery darkness of my womb.
Cell by cell you grew, unknown and longed for.
The gentle contractions of my uterus
break against your father's hands, his body anchors mine.
The waves become stronger, push me against the wall.
Your father with me in each breath,
dark blue eyes hold mine: be here, be here, be here.
I rock on the floor and moan low,
guttural sounds that echo around the womb and
call to you to come outside.
I find a ferocity I don't recognize as my own.
In a hospital room, push against a bed
no space between the waves, knocked down and
on top of me, gasp for breath
midwife, doula tell me something
a change of shift, new doctor, new doula
'too intense, too intense' but no one hears me
my mother beside me, her hand on my back

'let's get her to the birth pool'.
Sinking down, down into the birth pool,
I lean against your father,
take the doula's hand and surrender to her wisdom.
I push into each contraction for as long as I can,
then collapse into the water's strong arms.
Nothing left but the refusal to give up until you are with us.
From far away I hear my mother's voice,
'they're coming, they're coming!'
One more push and no burning just pressure released
as you swim out of my body and into the watery light,
the doctor catches you, brings you home to my breast.
In tired reverence I gaze at you.
Clothed in blood and shining amniotic fluid,
you look up at me with your father's face in miniature.
I hold the mystery of you against my heart, Jonah.

# Georgia Walker-Carter

*Georgia Walker-Carter is thirteen and lives in Lancashire with her mum and dad. When Georgia was eleven she attended the water birth of her sister Lola. Her parents gave this decision careful thought and felt it was important that Georgia was part of such a special moment for their family. Here Georgia tells her story.*

## The Birth of Lola!

It was a Saturday morning in January and I was fast asleep in bed, when all of a sudden my dad came and woke me up at 6.45am. He said to me, 'It's time to get ready, your mum's in labour'. My heart was thumping and I ran into my mum and dad's room and said to them, 'No you're not!' 'Yes she is', replied my dad. I really didn't believe them at first but when my dad told me to hurry and get ready, and I saw my mum sat on her bed taking deep breaths and concentrating, I was shocked but excited! I knew this was really it.

I collected my Nintendo DS and put on some comfortable clothing for the journey. When we were all ready to go and we had the hospital bags, we got in the car, but my dad had to defrost it first and began scraping the windows. Before we knew it, we were off to the birth centre. I sat quietly in the back of the car, looking outside whilst listening to my mum continue with her deep breathing in the front. As we got closer and closer to the birth centre, I remember feeling slightly nervous about what was going to happen next, but curious as to whether I was soon going to have a baby brother or sister.

At approximately 8.30am, we arrived at the birth centre. It

was a glorious sunny, but frosty morning. I helped my mum get out of the car whilst my dad brought in her hospital notes and bag. We walked to the main entrance of the birth centre and I rang the bell. I felt the vibration go through me with nerves! A nice woman came and answered the door and welcomed us into a private room. She then went and collected another midwife who introduced herself as Karen. Me and my dad sat on some chairs opposite a bed as my mum slowly climbed up onto it. Karen examined her to see how many centimetres dilated she was. She said she was four centimetres dilated and was definitely in labour. My dad and I therefore went back to the car to collect the rest of the bags while Karen helped my mum move across the corridor into a birthing room. It was a huge room with a bathroom, a bed, a water pool at one end and a garden/patio area outside the French doors. It was lovely.

As we entered the room, one of the midwives started running the water pool with hot soothing water. I put all the hospital bags down by some chairs at the end of the bed whilst my mum was putting her bikini top on. I watched as Karen helped my mum step carefully into the pool. I decided to go back to the car to get my iPod because I thought my mum might want to listen to some music while in labour. When I returned from the car my mum was leant against the edge of the pool, on her knees, swaying gently from side to side in the water, with her eyes shut. My dad was sat on a chair, by the pool, facing my mum and rubbing her back.

I went and put the iPod on the docking station on a little cabinet and asked my mum if she wanted the music on, but it was a very definite 'No' from her! I sat on the chair over by the bed, watching my mum, quietly and patiently. I remember thinking that the noises she was making were amusing. My point of view was that she sounded like a cow and an aeroplane. She was very loud! Altogether, she was in the water pool for about an hour and twenty minutes and during that time I was just sat in the chair the whole time, watching eagerly.

Finally it came to the point where my mum started pushing. Originally I told my mum that I wanted to go to the lounge to watch TV when she was pushing the baby out, but now it was really happening and I was really excited, so I went over to the pool and watched for the rest of the birth! It was amazing! I stood at the edge of the pool, next to the other midwife named Lisa, at the back of my mum. I could see the baby's head slowly appearing. Then the face became visible – I was fascinated! Then the rest of the baby's body emerged and its little legs were crossed. Lisa then leant forward and put her hands underneath the baby's head, in the water and gently pushed the baby forward towards Karen, the other midwife, who helped my mum pick the baby up out of the water and straight onto my mum's chest. My mum sat back in the water and Karen said, 'Congratulations, you've got a little girl, but I don't think she's that little! I think she'll be about 9lb!'

At this point I walked round to my dad, at the front of the pool, and burst into tears against his chest with happiness. I felt overwhelmed with joy! Me and my dad then went and stood over by my mum and had some pictures taken by Karen. After a few moments Lisa came and wrapped my baby sister in a towel and took her over to a little cot.

Whilst the midwives helped my mum get out of the pool and over to the bed, I stood next to my little sister in the cot, stroking her soft skin and admiring her. I was over the moon! The midwives helped my mum as she pushed out the placenta while I stayed with my new baby sister.

Then came the moment when they weighed the baby – she didn't seem to like this bit as she was crying – but she weighed 9lb 7oz!

Lisa then did lots of different checks on her. Once we knew everything was OK with the baby, my dad carried her over to my mum to have her first breastfeed. Once my sister had finished feeding, I then had my first cuddle with her. At first I was really stiff and nervous as I hadn't ever held a newborn baby before and didn't know how to hold her, but in the end I got the hang of it and became more relaxed. I loved cuddling her and caring for her throughout the rest of the day.

We decided to name her Lola Rose. The birth of my little sister was the best experience I've ever had and I will remember it for the rest of my life. I can't wait for Lola to grow up so I can tell her all about her birth.

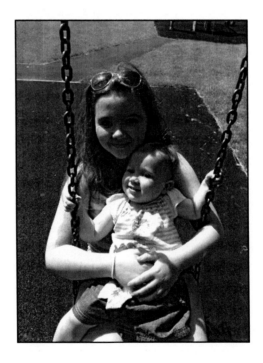

# Maggie Howell

*Maggie Howell is a birth expert, mother of five and a leading voice against the culture of fear that surrounds birth. In this story, she describes how she discovered the benefits of hypnosis for birth first-hand when she delivered her first child at home, in water and without so much as a paracetamol. She went on to use hypnosis in all of her subsequent births, and to develop Natal Hypnotherapy, now a leading provider of hypnosis for childbirth in the UK.*

## Joseph's Day

'Ohhh, my labour was 52 hours of sheer agony', 'All my good intentions went out the window – I begged for an epidural', 'I could not take any more so opted for a caesarean', 'You will never feel pain like it'. These were some of the experiences I heard when I proudly and excitedly announced I was pregnant. The more I listened to them and the more I read about similar birth stories in the pregnancy magazines, the more I was resolved not to have the same story to tell. I had always believed that birth was entirely natural, with our bodies specifically designed for it, and not a medical process in which intervention has become the norm.

To back this up, I had had two strong influential experiences about birth. The first came from my own childhood in Kenya where I had often heard the classic stories of women giving birth in bushes and then carrying on with their work. The second came from witnessing animals give birth. The proportion in size of their young to their birth canal is similar to humans and yet they are able to give birth with very little fuss and without the apparent pain that women often appear to have or drugs and intervention to deal with this. We know that animals can feel pain – so somehow animals are able to control their pain far better than humans during labour.

My thoughts about hypnosis and 'mind over matter' really began when a good friend gave birth in a small barn next to her house. It was her first baby and was technically a difficult birth – with a four-hour second stage! What really struck me was that she had not felt the need for any painkillers, as with each contraction her partner would describe somewhere or something they had done together. Effectively her mind was focusing on something other than the 'pain'. It was my husband who suggested going on a self-hypnosis course, as he in the past had used hypnosis to help with a variety of things. I was a little skeptical in the beginning, but decided that it could only help as I was determined to have a natural home birth.

I went on a two-day course when I was six months pregnant. I was the only pregnant woman on the course – the others were there for a whole variety of reasons from fear of public speaking, to giving up smoking, to stress relief. Prior to the course my only real experience of hypnosis was watching a stage hypnotist make people act like chickens and eat raw onions. I therefore assumed that there was something mystical about it and that I would close my eyes and be put in a semi-conscious state in which my all problems would be solved. However, after the first few times I doubted I had been hypnotised as I just felt very relaxed and was fully aware of my surroundings. As I discovered – that is exactly what hypnosis is! There is nothing magical about it. It is simply being in a daydream rather than in a conscious state. It is the same as when you realise that even though you have been driving your car carefully, you can't actually remember most of the journey. In hypnosis, you are having a chat with your subconscious, while your conscious mind is fully aware of what you are doing.

Over the next few weeks I wrote my self-hypnosis script or 'programme' for my vision of a positive birth. It included loads of triggers for relaxation, such as every time I had a contraction I would feel more and more relaxed, every time my husband held my hand I would feel more and more comfortable, and so on. I envisaged every last detail including my cervix opening, my baby feeling comfortable and safe, my muscles expanding, and holding my baby in my arms. Once I was happy with the programme I recorded it onto tape with some soothing music in the background. During the last six weeks I took myself into hypnosis every day and listened to the programme I had recorded on my tape recorder. The visualisation was so strong that I would often come out of hypnosis in tears, as if I had actually been through the experience of holding my precious baby. As the day came closer, I got more and more excited and was really looking forward to the birth. I was so keen to find out if the hypnosis would work and, in a way, to show others who had doubted what I was doing that I really could have a wonderful birth.

My first contraction finally came a few days after my due date at 10pm whilst eating dinner in a French restaurant. I had planned for a home water birth and so we excitedly returned to our house. Since the initial contractions were mild we caught some rest and then at 2.30am things really started to happen. We got everything ready for the birth – we lit a huge fire and lots of candles, made a nutritious milkshake and pots of raspberry leaf and nettle tea, and put on the soft music as we began what turned out to be a very long labour. I felt so calm and in control and was so sure that the hypnosis was going to work. Unfortunately my midwife, who had been really supportive of my hypnosis, was unable to attend the birth and so another midwife, a complete stranger, turned up to take care of me. She had never been with anyone who had used hypnosis and was obviously a bit skeptical, insisting that she had gas and air if I needed it. However, in my notes, which I read afterwards, she kept commenting on how relaxed, in control and calm I was.

I decided to leave it as long as possible before I got in the water and so spent many hours just relaxing on the birth ball. Being a first labour it took a very long time and after being at 5cm for more than three hours I decided to get in the pool to see if that helped things along. I will never forget the amazing feeling as I lowered myself into the warm water – it was magical. I felt so supported, safe, calm and at ease. Even though the contractions had been completely manageable until that point, once in the water they actually began to feel pleasurable and I began to look forward to each one, which was such an empowering feeling. I remember feeling that when in the water, no one could come into my space, and that felt really special.

I can truly say that until the last quarter of an hour I had absolutely no need for any painkillers and my breathing and dreamlike state kept me completely in control. My second midwife arrived after about six hours and did not actually hear me speak for three hours, even though my contractions were three minutes apart. My husband would occasionally ask where I was, to which I apparently replied 'away with the fairies' or 'on a beach' – these were images I had used in my hypnosis.

When I was finally fully dilated my midwife checked the baby's heartbeat just before I started to push. Very calmly she told us that his heartbeat had dropped substantially and that I would need to give birth out of the water. She knew we had to deliver the baby really quickly and suggested that I had an episiotomy⁺. This was the first time I felt real pain. I feel that there were two main reasons for it – firstly that I had not built this into my hypnosis programme, and secondly that I needed the adrenaline from the pain to push my baby out in the shortest possible time. The power and energy I felt was quite remarkable so I believe that the pain really helped me to ensure my son was born safely. Unbelievably Joseph was born just four minutes later. He was absolutely fine and within a minute took his first breath, coughed slightly and then looked up at me with calm blue eyes. He did not cry out or seem distressed in any way. We massaged him gently and put him straight on my breast, where he latched on immediately for his first drink. All those who came in contact with him commented on how calm and alert he was. I am sure this was partly due to my constant communication with him in utero and my continual reassurance during the birth that he was safe and soon to have a wonderful cuddle with his parents.

*When you see water in a stream*
*you say: oh, this is stream water;*
*When you see water in the river*
*you say: oh, this is water of the river;*
*When you see ocean water*
*you say: This is the ocean's water!*
*But actually water is always only itself*
*and does not belong*
*to any of these containers*
*though it creates them.*
*And so it is with you.*

**Alice Walker**

# Joanna Storey

*Joanna Storey chose to have her first baby at home, as she felt this would help her to feel in control of her labour. She also attended hypnobirthing classes and went on to have two home births. Joanna lives in Cheshire with her husband, two little ones and her dog. Here she and her mother Jackie give their different perspectives on her birth story.*

## Joanna's Story

I have had two water births at home and both were amazing. I was very aware of my mum's concern about me having a home birth and only using the water to assist with managing the birth. However, despite this I went ahead with the support of my husband, planned a home birth and attended hypnobirthing classes. I learnt so much from the hypnobirthing that I literally just breathed my way through both labours, staying focused, relaxed and calm and using cues (certain smells and music) to promote that relaxation.

I used the birthing pool to birth both my babies, getting in the water thirty-five minutes before my son was born and just five minutes before my daughter was born. The midwives at my daughter's birth tried to stop me from getting in the pool as they did not think the temperature was quite right – according to a textbook*. We quickly added kettles of water and I was in there like a shot as my baby was definitely ready to be born! I had the amazing experience of delivering both of my babies myself in the water, and my husband was also able to help receive them into our hands before putting them straight to my chest.

The pool created a sacred space for me and my baby to meet. A space that midwives could not enter and that they could not intervene in, until we were ready to get out of the pool. Be it in hospital or at home, I would not want to birth a baby in any other way again than in water.

# Jackie's Story

When my daughter Joanna first told me of her intention to have her baby at home, I felt very concerned. I had watched her suffer with severe migraine headaches and seen the impact that this had had on her. I remember thinking, 'If she can't cope with migraine there is no way she will cope with labouring at home with no pain relief'. Being a mother of five I knew the 'joys' of labouring and I personally could not imagine going through this away from a hospital environment and all that this affords. I didn't want to discourage her with all my tales of woe, however – my concerns were high. Joanna told me about 'hypnobirthing' and about the process of relaxing through the different stages. 'Relaxing, now that's a new one on me', I thought. Who ever heard of relaxing through labour?!

Well all I can say is, why didn't I know about hypnobirthing when I was having my children? Joanna gave me the privilege of inviting me into her most precious moment in life, and allowed me to be present while she brought our grandchild into the world. It was incredible. I walked into the room as she approached the second stage of labour. The atmosphere was so peaceful as the candles gently burned and the music played. Joanna was busy concentrating on her breathing as her body worked through each contraction. The moment felt so sacred. We quietly spoke during the rest periods and I stepped back as she breathed through the contractions. It was just awesome.

Joanna's waters broke and she transitioned into the pool. Pure delight lit up in her face instead of the fear and dread I had so often seen during the episodes of migraine. Four big pushes and our grandchild entered the world. There was absolutely no comparison between what I was seeing and my own experience of childbirth. If I wasn't 52, I'd go back and do it all again.

*The river is flowing, flowing and growing*
*The river is flowing, back to the sea*
*Mother Earth carry me*
*Your child I will always be*
*Mother Earth carry me*
*Back to the sea.*

**Pagan chant**

# Gauri Lowe

*Gauri Lowe is a medical doctor working in women's health. Her two home births in South Africa were deeply empowering life-changing moments directing her to dedicate her professional life to provide deep nurturing support to pregnant women. She lives in Cape Town with her two sons and husband.*

## From Medical School to Water Birth

About seventeen years ago I started my path into the vast world of healthcare. I began my medical studies after high school, with high aspirations of 'helping people heal'. Disillusioned with the teachings and paradigms taught at medical school, I became involved in a then young world of natural, traditional and holistic approaches to healing our bodies and minds.

I took some time away from my studies to find the answers to my yearning questions. I wanted to go deeper... I wanted to understand what causes disease beyond the physical matter of bodies and chemicals, the connection between mind and emotion, disease and healing. I came across an ancient practical spirituality which satisfied my personal hunger and my healing questions. So I stayed, studied, travelled, taught and lived that world completely for seven years.

Then my dormant desire for healing roused and reignited. With an absolute but unexplainable conviction I returned to my medical studies. For years I continued in a world which felt in so many ways wrong, harsh, missing the point – but fascinating, real and dynamic. My holistic interest remained true and a friend and I created the 'Complementary Medicine Society' at medical school. We hosted talks and exposures to alternate, natural and holistic healing for medical students and staff.

By my third year of medicine I was married, in love and happily pregnant.

Little did I know how this was going to swerve my natural medical approaches yet again! I had little practical training in birth at this point but I had unquestionable faith that I wanted to birth at home and not go near a hospital, which seemed alien and scary to me. I learned more about creating the fourth stage of labour as calm, quiet, dimly lit and serene for the baby to adjust to the new and big world outside. I knew that birth was about the parents meeting and welcoming the baby into the world.

I had a private midwife and six weeks after my final term exams I had a serene, undisturbed, life-changing home birth during one winter night in our small suburban flat.

And that was another turning point.

I had tasted conscious birth.

Lochan was born as headstrong and present as he still is. And afterwards we snuggled into my bed, as my husband served the best breakfast I have ever tasted in my life!

I felt like I had connected with something so sacred and sublime. I felt like I had gone through a passageway to motherhood shared by all mothers across species. I felt one with the organic pulse of Mother Nature at her most intense, rawest, purest self.

And I began to devour the research, finding a giant world supporting and explaining why gentle conscious birth forms an important part of creating peaceful communities one birth at a time.

I began to realise that birth was a most essential, wonderful ingredient available to all as a lovely start to life and parenting.

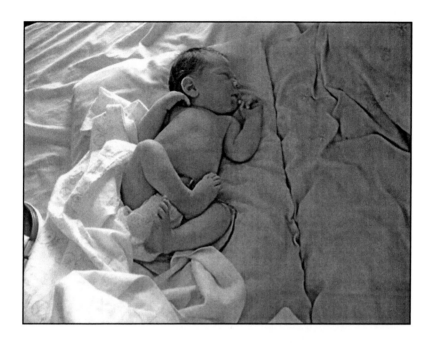

The realisation and conviction of this knowledge came with challenges as I studied and practised in a medical, high turnover, often high-risk environment, with doctors unaware of the jewels pregnancy and birth hold.

From a positive perspective I have grown to appreciate the role of medical intervention when it is properly indicated. With a more complete view of medicine, I still appreciate supporting and empowering women in pregnancy and birth as an essential part of primary health care. It is prevention at its primal roots – as every person starts off being a foetus and then born.

There is abundant research now supporting the essential effects of pregnancy, birth and parenting on individuals and communities. The fields include psychological, anthropological, physical, neuro-chemical, developmental, emotional and histori-cal! It is fascinating, widespread and very real. The more effort and education we can surmount to allow an awareness and a practice of gentle and conscious pregnancy, birth and parenting the more we can spread a culture of love, empathy and awareness.

# The Birth of Shyam

The thing about giving birth is that you have to be very open. The energy is very powerful and opens you up. And we need to let that energy flow through and open us. This takes a huge surrender. Anything tense or withholding causes a blockage. It also causes pain as the natural driving energy is to be soft and open and flowing.

My baby and I guided my whole labour. From when my water broke and I resumed resting in bed – waiting and wondering when the contractions would start. My first baby also started like this but it was night time and the contractions built slowly as we slept in bed in between (a bit in denial).

Now, after delivering and witnessing many hospital deliveries as a doctor, observing and doing several home births, reading, learning and educating people about natural conscious gentle birth – I was waiting for my own to begin. The huge organic event that occurs ending each pregnancy – the birth of my second child that would forever from that time – change our family to four, my seven-year-old son to older brother.

They niggled slowly and as my husband and son set up the birth pool I came upstairs, the contractions calling for my focused attention as they mounted. I curled up in bed as my son took to dusting around me ('cleaning up his office') and drew a picture of the pond next door.

There was no conscious boundary or change but the contractions had become more consuming and I was within them as they were within me.

I screamed in my labour. The contractions were opening

me and my baby was navigating his own descent. I could feel it from the inside out. I started off with harmonic deep basal 'oooooohhhhhssss'. These felt very good and natural and helped to guide the energy through and out of me. I closed my eyes most of the time as I let the energy flow in and through and then relax in between contractions. My closed eyes allowed me to be in my own cocoon.

After about forty-five minutes of this I got into the water. When I was in the water I opened my eyes only to reposition myself, to grasp the handle, to hang over the side. And at one point I opened my eyes as my midwife said 'Look at me. You can do this'. Other than that my eyes stayed closed and I was in this dance. The pains rose and my voice rose – carrying the pain of the contractions through me and out. And then when the intensity increased and I felt pain I started shouting or screaming. I had to get it out and it was so intense I had to be more intense and forceful.

My mother had died suddenly during my pregnancy. She was too young to die and she got sick and we visited her for ten days in hospital knowing she would never recover from her disabling stroke, leaving her unable to move or communicate besides eye movement. My baby was finishing his first trimester. He was twelve weeks in utero when she died. And we mourned together and went to the funeral together and continued the grieving together as he was within me.

I screamed in my labour to release this terrible emotional pain, grief and loss. I finally let it out as my baby had to move through my blockages to enter this world. And this pain had definitely nestled in some blockages in my system. So I screamed at the unfairness of it and I screamed that my son would never experience his grandmother, who was the most loving, caring, wonderful grandmother to his brother. But it probably just looked like I was screaming with each contraction.

This same surrender we find in spiritual truths. Surrendering to something much bigger and more awesome than you... is what we have to do in birth. You really can't hold onto anything. This perfect natural most powerful pure raw energy moves you and demands you move with it.

The most amazing part for me was pushing my baby out. My body started pushing so we knew it was time. There had been no examinations at all. I could feel I was opening up. And then when the pushing started I knew that was time. The pain of the contractions changed. My body surged with the pushes and I could feel my baby's head crowning.

With my breath and hand (two senses – touch and my inner sense of pain and burning) I controlled the crowning of my baby's head. In this way the stretching was gradual – and I birthed intact. I felt his head rotate. I caught him as his body slipped out of mine. I raised him to my chest. And then I enjoyed the huge relief and release of birth. And he cried as we held each

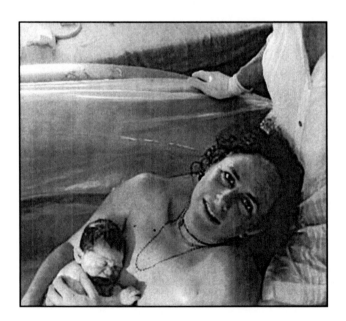

other. Accepting and embracing our meeting. The meeting of my second child that I had been dreaming of for years, that I had been praying for and meditating on for so long and that I had been nurturing for months.

## Lotus Birth

I never thought or planned a lotus birth. Delayed cord clamping made sense. But keeping the baby attached to the placenta, not cutting the cord at all – just letting it separate when it was ready – this was never something that particularly appealed to me. Probably as I am a vegetarian and a medical doctor! I didn't want to hang on to the placenta and I needed a bit more 'evidence/reason' to keep it attached.

On asking my midwife the reasons for lotus birth – as the placenta of course is no longer nutritive or physically supportive – the reply made sense. 'It is spiritual.' It symbolises the natural separation of the baby as separate from its life source – marking the fourth stage.

'Lotus Birth is a call to pay attention to the natural physiological process. Its practice, through witnessing, restores faith in the natural order. Lotus Birth extends the birth time into the sacred days that follow and enables baby, mother and father and all family members to pause, reflect and engage in nature's conduct. Lotus Birth is a call to return to the rhythms of nature, to witness the natural order and to the experience of not doing, just being.' (*Lotus Birth*, by Rachana Shivam)

So I thought I would see how we felt at the time. After our quick and intense but wonderful and beautiful and empowering water birth, I remember feeling the cord pulsating at one point – before the placenta was delivered. Holding on to my baby and feeling the cord still pulsating – quite a thought!

And then it seemed right to keep it attached. And then it continued to seem right. Actually very right. I could see how this little one was interacting with it, used to it and part of it. His hand would fall on it. His foot would rest on it. We just moved it left or right of him to feed or care for him. We bathed him and put the plastic bucket with the placenta in in the bath too. We emptied out the fluid everyday and added more salt to cover it. It never smelled. We kept the umbilicus clean as normal. And we watched the cord become hardened overnight and then harder and brittle.

On the morning of day five, the cord separated naturally. And it was a special moment! It did feel like the time had come and today was his separation day or independence day! It felt momentous and it happened when he was ready.

We dug a hole for it, planted the placenta with the cord stretching upwards in a spiral and placed our plant on top of it.

I am so happy we spontaneously did the lotus birth. It has felt very right – organic and part of a natural birth process that I hadn't been so aware of before. My baby has been calm, content, quiet and very peaceful, having spent the first few days of his life with his placenta still attached.

# Jenn Clegg

*Jenn Clegg's first birth was a caesarean section for a breech presenting baby at 38 weeks. With her second pregnancy she wanted a home birth, but her plans seemed threatened when she discovered this baby was also breech. However, with support from an Independent Midwife, Jenn went on to birth her baby at home in water.*

## Jenn's Story

As soon as I found out I was pregnant I was of the mind that I would like a home birth, but knew that I would have a fight on my hands as I had had a previous caesarean section for a breech presenting baby. I spoke to an NHS midwife about my thoughts of a home VBAC, and a look of horror appeared over her face followed by many negative comments. From her reaction, I knew I wouldn't be supported by the NHS. My husband James and I discussed my situation with friends and family — many of them said to get on with things and that it doesn't matter how bad the birth is because you will forget all the pain when you hold your baby. I wouldn't accept this because I wanted to look back at the birth of my baby as a highlight of my life, not something I was desperate to forget.

After getting upset and stressed that I wasn't being heard, a friend recommended an Independent Midwife* called Debs. We gave Debs a call and within five minutes I knew that I had to have her as my midwife because she was so positive about birth. From then on I felt so relaxed and began to enjoy being pregnant. Debs gave me a wealth of information and I felt totally empowered by the decisions I was making about my pregnancy.

At about 26 weeks I joined a hypnobirthing course. I had a real fear of the head crowning and needed help to over come this. Hypnobirthing was a great technique but I was still scared. I continued to practise my breathing technique every night, hoping my fear would eventually disappear because I was excited about meeting my baby.

At 37 weeks Debs came to do an antenatal check and I told her I was sure I could feel a head under my ribs. Debs palpated and sure enough the baby was breech. I did not feel panicked – if anything I was quite excited. Debs was still happy to carry on planning a home birth with me. I went for a scan to confirm the breech position, but this got the obstetric team in a spin and I was booked for a c-section there and then. I just went with it knowing damn well I wasn't having it – I simply couldn't be bothered with the fight of explaining my choices. Once home I rang to cancel: much easier!

I went home and began to research like crazy. My instinct was saying all was well but I needed to know more. Fortunately Debs had encouraged me to read a few books already because I was at a higher risk of carrying a breech baby because of my previous breech. I began my web search with AIMS* and took it from there. The more I read the more I was reassured that birthing a breech baby is absolutely possible. I did try to get the baby to change position with reflexology and osteopathy. James even talked, played music and shone a light low down on my bump in the hope that baby would go and investigate, but baby stayed put.

I had a lengthy appointment with Debs, who went through the birth process of a breech baby with a doll and pelvis and explained the risks that are associated with breech births. She explained the manoeuvres they might use if difficulties arose. Debs was confident and experienced, which gave me confidence.

A second midwife would have to attend the birth due to the increased risks, so an appointment was made to meet Michelle.

For the next week I carried on researching like crazy. *Breech Birth* by Benna Waites and Anthony Craib and the AIMS book *Breech Birth* were two books I read over and over. They gave me a wealth of information as well as providing me with further reading. The more I read the more I was reassured and fascinated that breech births were viewed as such a problem.

I met with Michelle at my next antenatal appointment and she, just like Debs, was amazing and I was pleased she was now involved in my care. From this appointment I realised I had made my decision to birth my baby at home. I had researched the risks of a VBAC and breech birth and I felt birthing at home was the right choice for me. So I put all books and articles away and looked forward to birthing day. This was not to happen for another two weeks.

On 6 September I woke up to some mild contractions and went into complete denial and set out on a day trip. After ten minutes in the car I was very uncomfortable being restricted by the seat belt so we headed home!

Once home all I wanted was to be in water but felt I should hold off so I compromised and went in the shower. At 9am we contacted Debs to let her know things were happening. By 10.30am I felt I needed her with me so I asked her to attend and I got in the pool. The contractions felt completely different to what I was expecting and I was amazed at how well the hypnobirthing techniques were working. Debs and Michelle arrived and I felt reassured and relaxed that everything was in place. It was quiet and calm and I just breathed my way through the contractions.

At about half past three things seemed to step up a gear. I began to struggle and asked to be examined. Debs reassured me all was going well but the contractions had become really strong and I really wanted to know if I was getting somewhere, so insisted on a vaginal examination. I was delighted when Debs said I was 9cm and it gave me the strength and positivity to carry on. Baby was still high so I stayed out of the pool to see if gravity would help. One and a half hours later I needed the relief of the pool so I got back in and it was a much welcomed comfort to be back in the water. The gas and air was helping me greatly but supplies were becoming low so Debs contacted the local hospital and arranged for more cylinders to be delivered. I was so relieved by this as the gas and air had become what felt like my lifeline!

There was a very distinct point when I had a contraction and all of a sudden I stopped breathing through it and held my breath. After spending the whole labour with my eyes closed they shot open and I remember looking at Debs and screaming silently 'I don't want to do this bit, I am terrified'. Debs gave me a reassuring nod and told me to go with it. I carried on breathing as much as possible and tried so hard to stay relaxed, but I was fighting my instinct as much as I could. The contractions became very expulsive and I went deep within myself and just tried to listen to my body. Debs explained that I was trying to get on all fours (often seen in a physiological breech birth), but that the height of the water was restricting me so I got out of the pool. I was still resisting the urge to push and it was at this stage I said to myself, 'This baby has got to come out, get on with it'! The next push I gave it everything I had and rumping (as crowning is called in a breech birth), happened very quickly, followed by the body. The relief of the pressure was immense. Two sharp sensations happened which were the legs releasing, I remember looking through my legs and seeing a little body! Then there were a few sharp uncomfortable movements as the baby wriggled its arms out.

My contractions at this point had stopped. Debs could see no chin on the chest so examined me and found the head to be extended. An ambulance was called and Debs started manoeuvres to birth the baby. No movement was felt so I was encouraged to change position and Michelle tried nipple stimulation to get contractions coming. Michelle and James helped me to stand, Debs attempted head flexion, movement was felt, I was encouraged to push. Suddenly baby was born, immediately followed by the placenta! I remember looking down to see baby and being shocked to see the placenta. Debs was right behind me resuscitating baby and it was only at this point that I felt any kind of worry or panic because everything had remained calm and quiet. I remember looking at Debs with my baby – the baby opening his eyes – Michelle telling me there was a heartbeat. I was reassured by this and felt all would be OK. I glanced across at James who looked worried. I heard a noise behind me and there was an ambulance crew, which really shocked me because I was completely unaware they had been called, never mind arrived. Debs said to get ready to go to hospital but my legs wouldn't work; James literally had to pick me up and dress me. My body had nothing else to give. Debs at this stage was still resuscitating the baby, but he was making efforts to breathe for himself and his colour and tone had improved. Ten minutes after birth we were in the ambulance on our way to hospital and baby was breathing independently.

Once at the hospital we were shown to a room and I finally got to hold my baby. He opened his eyes and looked straight at me, it felt amazing. We stayed there undisturbed for a couple of hours. I have to say the NHS midwife who looked after us was lovely as I was very nervous about being judged. We made our phone calls and had something to eat. Baby had some colostrum* hand-expressed into his mouth. Everything was very relaxed and settled. After a while I had a shower and got ready to be transferred to the postnatal ward. Once on the ward baby was skin-to-skin, and that was how we stayed all night with me gazing at him and expressing colostrum into him every so often. It was far from perfect because I really wanted to be in my bed with my husband and baby, and I was on my own in a single hospital bed. However, I still feel like I had the most exhilarating experience of my life.

I feel completely liberated by my birth experience. I am so pleased I had Debs and Michelle around me as they just seemed to know when to encourage me, when to have a laugh and when to leave me to it. I never felt out of control even when things became difficult at the end. At no point did I feel over-whelmed – I was fully debriefed and I completely understood what happened. I look back so fondly at my birth experience and can't wait to do it again!

# Rachel Barber

*Rachel Barber had her firstborn in hospital and found the experience to be rather clinical. In spite of some anxiety and fear of the unknown, she chose a birth centre water birth for her second. Here, she and her husband Charley take turns to recall the fantastic experience and the rather large addition to the family! Rachel and Charley live near Accrington with their two adorable children.*

## Rachel's Story

*Monday: 11 days overdue!*

After several sweeps and shows* (and numerous nesting moments making sure everything was spotless) I had somewhat reluctantly resigned myself to the possibility that I was going to be induced*.

I woke up in the morning, having sent my husband back to work (some 180 miles away!) with no signs that 'this could be the day'. Maisy (our beautiful little girl, age four) was at home with me and we were having a lazy morning. Maisy wanted to stay in bed and watch TV, which was fine by me! I then decided to take the opportunity to enjoy a shower, after which I was getting dressed and suddenly felt a little trickle. I didn't really think anything of it until I went to the toilet and noticed that my underwear was wet through. I had been told that amniotic fluid has a distinct smell to it and it was then I knew that my waters were leaking. I didn't make a fuss and calmly said to Maisy that 'Mummy just has to make a phone call'.

I rang the birth centre and explained what had happened

and they asked me to pop in for an examination. Luckily I had already spoken to my parents that morning and arranged for them to come over so that Maisy could have some time with Grandad, and my mum and I could nip out to take my wedding, engagement and eternity rings to be cleaned – another nesting moment! When my parents arrived I quietly explained to them at the door what was happening as I didn't want to alarm Maisy. At this point I hadn't mentioned anything to my husband either! I discreetly put the bags I had prepared in the car and Mum and I set off to the birth centre.

On arrival I was getting out of the car and noticed that the trickle had turned into a bigger trickle. We didn't have to wait long and we were taken to a consultation room where the midwife confirmed that my waters were leaking and labour could happen at any time, although at this point I wasn't having any pains. As soon as I stood up from the bed there was a 'gush' and I was wet through, an exciting but awkward moment! The midwife explained the procedure that if nothing had happened within the next 24 hours an appointment would have to be made for me to be induced at the hospital, due to risk of infection. I also had to take my temperature every four hours. The phone call was made to my husband and he promptly made the journey back home.

Mum and I made our way back home. My Dad obviously hadn't heard me properly when we arrived and he said, 'You've been a long time to get your rings cleaned!' which made me laugh!

We kept Maisy occupied playing games and colouring until my husband Charley arrived home. All the while I was rocking forwards and backwards and moving around a lot to try and progress things and get the baby in a good position.

Around 5pm Daddy arrived and had some time with Maisy before she went for a 'sleep over' to Grandma and Grandad's, which she was excited about.

Charley and I decided to watch the Ayrton Senna DVD – we are both Formula One fans – after which I took my temperature and headed to bed... still no pains! During the night Charley woke me to take my temperature and was really looking after me.

## Tuesday

At 6am the pains started! I got in the bath and listened to the Adele album – it was just what I needed! By the time I was getting out of the bath the pains were more regular and intense – but not enough to stop me enjoying a coffee! I phoned the birthing centre and they asked for me to hold out until contractions were five minutes apart and lasting more than a minute – that didn't take long and by 8am we were on our way.

On arrival, having walked from the car park, the contractions were relentless and we were promptly greeted by Joan (our midwife) and Michael (a student doctor). As the contractions were coming so regularly we had to be quick with the internal examination – I was 5cm dilated and I remember Joan saying that this baby was going to be here soon!

Joan asked me if I wanted to try the birthing pool – something I had always been apprehensive about. I explained that I was nervous about this but agreed to give it a go, fully supported by Charley – and what a relief it was! As soon as I entered the pool I was so much more relaxed and the warm water was so lovely. I tried the gas and air but really didn't want anything in my mouth and I just decided to get 'in the zone', close my eyes and breathe myself through it!

I kept asking for reassurance from my husband and Joan and I got it. I do remember at one point saying I wanted to get out, knowing full well that I wasn't going anywhere because the water was providing so much support and comfort.

After around an hour in the pool I suddenly felt the need to push and Joan quickly sent for the second midwife, Jessica (who I politely had to tell not to stroke my hand!). I had a few puffs of the gas and air whilst pushing (but nowhere near the amount I consumed whilst having Maisy!). I had got myself into a good position to deliver, it didn't seem long and I was in the final stages. With one last push at 10.49am our bouncing baby boy was born (still in his sac). He was absolutely beautiful, there were tears of joy, and Charley was thrilled to be able to cut the cord.

Now at that point we knew he was big, but it wasn't until Jessica put him on the scales that we realised how big... a whopping 11lb 13oz, delivered naturally, in the water with absolutely no intervention. The biggest baby to date to be born there!

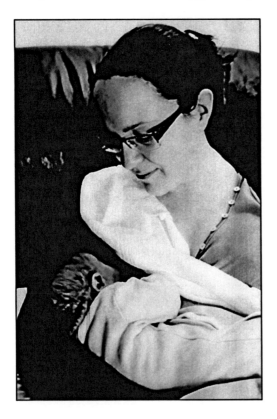

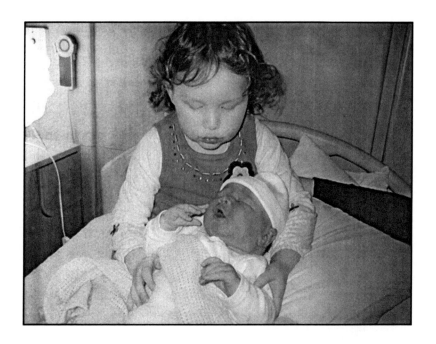

We were left to enjoy Noah and didn't feel rushed at all to move to the rest area, although when this time came I could see that Maisy had arrived with Mum and Dad and was patiently waiting to meet her little brother. The door opened, I saw her, and she saw me and promptly ran into my arms, a special moment I will always treasure (and which also made the receptionist cry!). After a couple of hours rest, we all headed back home, our family complete.

I honestly could wax lyrical about the whole experience and I am so pleased to have chosen Blackburn Birthing Centre and a water birth to have our baby boy. I found Maisy's birth harder and the surroundings very clinical in hospital, whereas at the birthing centre I was so relaxed – it really felt like 'home'. Water births are amazing and I would recommend them to anyone who is fortunate enough to be offered one.

Now for number 3????

# Charley's Story

I'm the lucky father of two very beautiful children; Maisy aged five, and Noah, aged ten months. I also have an amazing wife – Rachel, and this is my account of how Noah was delivered into the world.

Rachel – my wife – was eight days overdue, and I was home on the Friday night for the weekend after working away all week, hoping and praying that this would be the weekend for our baby to be born. Saturday and Sunday came and went with still no sign and I had to return to work early on the Monday morning. I had been at work for only half a day when I received a phone call from Rachel to say that her waters had broken, and that I should come home. She also said not to panic as she wasn't having any contractions and was with her mother at the birthing centre talking to a midwife. I panicked and began the drive home – not wanting to miss anything but still keeping within the speed limits was quite a tricky task!

Meanwhile the midwife sent Rachel home, with the explicit instructions to go to Burnley General Hospital at 11am for induction if there were still no signs of the baby arriving, but to come back to the Blackburn Birthing Centre if things should start happening sooner. I arrived home – in good time – and we packed Maisy off to Rachel's parents just in case we had to dash in the middle of the night. We calmly settled down for the evening, having supper and watching, of all things, a DVD about Ayrton Senna.

We both woke at 6am having had quite a good sleep, considering. I ran Rachel a bath and put some music on. I was downstairs making breakfast when Rachel called down saying that she was having contractions... yippee! By 8am the contractions were coming thick and fast, so we got in the car and made our ten-mile journey to the centre, in rush hour. We got there and Rachel had to use me for support to walk to the front door. We rang the bell to be let in by one of the midwives just as Rachel was having another contraction which stopped her in her tracks, and the midwife commented, 'We'll be getting you booked in then!'

They showed us to our room, by which time Rachel's contractions were coming very regularly and lasting more than a minute, almost like relentless waves, where a series of them would be bunched together, but Rachel was as calm as I'd ever seen her, she was in the zone, and ready for this baby, more than anything. We were asked if we'd like a water birth, which we did, so the large, purpose-built tub was filled, whilst the midwife and a student doctor carried out an examination. However this was proving a little difficult because the contractions were now so close together, Rachel could not relax enough for Joan to get 'access' for a proper exam. No matter, there was no turning back now, the tub was ready and Rachel scooted and shuffled across the room and climbed in, with my assistance of course.

'Not long now', said Joan. Rachel asked if the baby would be alright being born into water and Joan reassured her that babies are carried in fluid and don't draw their first breath straight away, that it was naturally safe, and that thousands of babies have been delivered this way.

So here we are – me sat on the outside of the tub and Rachel up to her chest in water – we're face to face, with Rachel's chin resting on the lip of the tub. She controlled her breathing as the contractions kept coming, and only had the odd toot on the gas and air, as she said it made her feel funny and she didn't like the taste. Rachel was offered other forms of pain relief but she felt that things were bearable for now and that she would soldier on. Joan was always there to offer words of encouragement and she involved me, letting me see the baby's head crowning with the use of a mirror on a stick placed in the water and angled strategically, so I could catch a glimpse of the head that had a smattering of dark hair – this was amazing.

Joan then made the call, time to push. A second midwife joined us. Rachel had her eyes closed, still controlling her own breathing, taking the odd gulp of gas and air, but really, really calm and like I say, in the zone. I was still knelt in front of her but not touching as I could see she was doing this and didn't want a fuss. In what seemed like a flash, our baby was born into the world at 10.49am. 'It's a boy', said Joan, 'and he's still in his sac'.

Now I'm not sure on the actual terminology, but he was basically born covered from head to toe in a transparent type membrane – apparently this is a sign of good fortune for the newly born baby. The membrane was removed from his face and Rachel looked up at me and asked pensively if he was ok and was he breathing? With the question came the answering cry from our bundle of joy: 'Yes', I said, 'He's fine'. The midwives asked if I'd like to cut the cord. I was welling up with happiness.

I helped Rachel out of the pool and onto the bed to birth the placenta. Whilst this was going on the boy was being weighed, and he's a big lad... '5.39 kilograms' says the midwife. 'OK', I say, 'What's that in old money?' '11lb 13oz', came the reply! Good God, he's a giant! We were later informed that he was the biggest baby ever born in the birthing centre – an accolade he holds to this day. We had no idea he was going to be that big; nothing showed on the scans or any of the checkups and to be honest, Rachel looked smaller carrying him than she did with Maisy (Maisy was 8lb 14oz), so it was all a bit of a surprise.

While Rachel had a 'few' stitches, I got acquainted with my brand new son, who, I might add, was as calm as his mummy, with almost a contented feel to him. I held him close to my

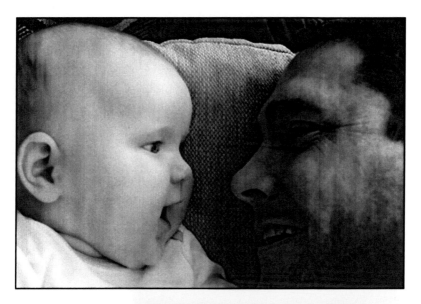

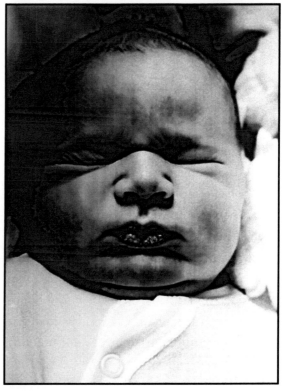

face and gently shushed him and he was as quiet as a mouse. After Rachel had been cleaned up by Joan, Noah was passed to Mummy for some vital skin-to-skin. This was special time for mother and baby, and I just had to stand back in awe and wonderment of the miracle that is childbirth, and at what my wife had achieved.

# Eleanor Copp

*Eleanor Copp qualified as a midwife in 1993. Her story describes how her own water birth, and the woman-centred care she received, ignited her passion to support women to feel similarly strong and empowered, and to listen to and trust their bodies. Eleanor lives in Somerset with her husband and children.*

## Eleanor's Stories

I started witnessing water births in my work as a midwife at Hillingdon Hospital in 1997, and was lucky enough to benefit from the great knowledge and wisdom of the then Head of Midwifery, Cass Nightingale. She was quiet, calm and supported amazing births in water; everything I saw her do was etched on my brain for posterity!

She was hands off the baby during the birth, and once the baby emerged into the water she would gently bring them to the surface to the mother.

I became quickly in love with supporting births in water, because the dynamic between mother and baby seemed more powerful, and their being in the water together was their space and not mine.

It did help, of course, that I had experienced my own water birth in 1996 in St Mary's, Paddington. My tutor from my midwifery training, Maureen, had supported me to have my second baby Harry in the pool, and it was a fantastic experience. I remember the things she said to me to this day, and so, on my return to work following maternity leave, my eyes and sentiments had been opened by a personal experience that had been wonderful.

My first son was born on my twenty-fifth birthday, and I remember thinking that my midwifery training had not prepared me at all for giving birth myself, as I had thought it would. The labour was about fifteen hours long, and he was born healthy and strong. I was overjoyed, repeating again and again 'My baby my baby my baby', as I held him for the first time in my arms. The labour was defined by lovely compassionate care from my friends, but also by things which hurt me: the interventions, specifically having the first internal exam, having a drip put in my hand and having a catheter put in my urethra.

Pregnant for the second time, and with the continuous support of my past tutor Maureen, I felt confidence in myself to plan to have this baby in the pool. As with my first son Freddie, my waters released in the morning in bed before I felt any contractions, but surprisingly early at 38 weeks. It was the day of my leaving do at work! My Mum travelled up from Somerset to London, arriving at 11pm, and we went off to Paddington, not because I was in active labour really but because we had a flat, space was tight and I was becoming a bit worried and impatient.

When we got there I wasn't doing much, contraction-wise, so I wandered around feeling some relief that I was there and so was Maureen, but some disappointment too that it was 'slow'.

The contractions got stronger and more powerful as the night wore on and I stared longingly at the pool. I got in around 5am, and found it immediately lovely. Lovely because of the warmth and water surrounding all of my body. I could move and time passed differently. Harry was born at 6.31am; my active labour was about four hours. I know that a second birth is often a very healing experience and certainly it was for me. I had no interventions through this labour, and held him in the pool for a while, then I got out of the pool with the cord still attached, and the placenta came out simply. This set the tone for my daughter's home birth three years later.

Harry was and remains very calm, unruffled and adorable. All my children have different personalities, but he is certainly less reactive than the other three, and in my mind that is in part due to his being born in water.

His birth was the catalyst for my future passion and confidence in this way of supporting births, which at the time was new and therefore rare. This personal experience has enabled me to replicate in my professional life the opportunity to birth in water for hundreds of women and their babies since then.

I have been present at so many wonderful births in the pool that are all memorable for totally different reasons. However, this one stands out in my memory; it was so moving I was left speechless.

A dad got in the pool with his partner who was in labour, she wanted him in there, and, although tentative, he wanted to support her and do as she asked. He got in, and found a position where he could hold her. He was sitting with his back against the pool side and she was leaning into him so that they were facing each other. He said he could feel the baby kicking and the expulsive movement of her womb during the contractions. She was burying her head in his chest and receiving bodily support by his physical presence and commitment of love.

The contact this baby had with both her parents in the later stages of labour was special. He said he could feel the bump getting lower – his knowledge of the descent of the baby was brilliant and so accurate. I trusted him with everything he said, especially when the baby's head became visible to me! This couple were so in tune with each other and their baby – it was special. Their intimacy and awareness of each other meant that this was truly a shared experience and I am sure this allowed their daughter to emerge smoothly. As the baby came towards me, I gently passed her through her mother's legs and brought her up in between her parents, and she looked at them. In the middle, as she had been, as she still was.

They were ecstatic. And I was in tears as usual.

# Ali Pember

*Ali Pember chose to have her first baby at her local birth centre but, due to midwife shortages, the unit was shut when she went into labour. However, she was still able to use a birthing pool on the hospital maternity ward and this, along with amazing support from her doula Jady and midwife Eleanor Copp (see previous story), led to a very positive birth experience. Ali lives with her daughter Clemmie and partner Bob in an old farmhouse in Somerset which they are renovating together.*

## Ali's Story

It was just over a week before my due date, but I had a sense that, because the baby was in the perfect position and her head was engaged, she could come at any time. I started to experience period-type pains on and off over a few days, and on Monday morning I got out of bed and felt a small trickle of waters breaking as I stood up. It wasn't a huge amount, so I realised it was probably just a tear, and that active labour could still be some way off.

Throughout my pregnancy I had learned to trust myself over things like the baby's growth being fine despite not measuring right for dates, and this was no different. I was determined not to contact the hospital only for them to put me up against the clock! I phoned my doula, Jady, and she was also reassuring. During the course of the day my waters continued to leak and I also began to see some mucus 'show'. I also had the period-type pains continually. I knew she was coming but I felt it was important to take my time at home, and again, this was a case of trusting my own intuition.

I managed to get some sleep on Monday night, but by Tuesday morning the pains were coming in more regular waves. I found that the best way of managing them was by making slow clockwise circles sitting on the birthing ball and taking long breaths, making a low humming sound on each of my out breaths. This was a pattern I stayed with for pretty much all of the first phase of labour, just increasing my focus as the pain grew stronger. Conveniently, I had an antenatal appointment already booked in with Jady for 11am and when she came, I was still able to talk through the contractions, so she left to get her birthing kit and Bob went to stock up on snacks as we weren't very prepared...

Of course, while I was on my own, the contractions decided to up the ante! Suddenly they required my full concentration through each build-up and peak of intensity. I was very inwardly focused, but I also wanted to have some emotional support. I called my mum at about 2pm and talked to her between contractions. Every time one came I had to hang up, work through it by breathing and rocking, and then call her back. We spoke on and off for about forty minutes, and mum said the contractions were coming about every ten minutes or so.

Bob came back and I asked him to phone the hospital. We spoke to Chrissy, the midwife from Malawi whom we had seen for our booking-in appointment at the Birth Centre, but I think the fact that I recognised her voice and sounded calm enough to talk meant that she thought I was not as far advanced in labour as I was. Unfortunately, we were told that it was not possible to go into the Birth Centre, so I knew, with some trepidation, that I would be on the main maternity ward.

I stayed at home for another couple of hours. I got really wobbly and shaky, which I thought was due to fatigue, but I now realise was most likely adrenaline kicking in at transition. Jady came back and started to prepare me to go to the hospital. First I had to get off the birthing ball, something I was very reluctant to do as I felt safe and secure sitting on it. She got me on my hands and knees and could see that I was moving into the second stage of labour. Somehow I managed to walk downstairs to the car with Bob and Jady's support. I remember dropping to my hands and knees on the ground in the front garden during the next contraction and feeling the grass under my hands. It felt good to be connected with the earth.

I leant over the backseat of the car and closed my eyes as we began the journey to the hospital down twisting country lanes. It felt like an eternity to get there, as I kept having very intense contractions, had less freedom of movement, and was trying to resist the urge to push. Jady massaged my lower back, which really helped. One of the worst sensations was actually pins and needles in my feet due to the position I was stuck in, so she also rubbed them to give me some relief!

We got to the hospital, and I was offered a wheelchair but chose to walk supported by Bob and Jady. Once again, I remember dropping on to all fours during a contraction, but this time on to the less forgiving surface of a hospital corridor. We made it into the birthing room on the maternity ward, which had a pool, and thankfully the midwife on duty was Eleanor Copp, so I felt relieved that we would be in good hands. She and Jady knew each other and had worked together before. I got up on the bed and Eleanor examined me internally. She was surprised to find that I was fully dilated. All that hard work and focus at home (and in the car!) had been worth it. She said the magic words, 'You can begin to push', but I didn't quite believe it, not knowing I had already gone through transition. I was expecting to get to a point where I felt that I couldn't go on, but that never happened.

I chose to get into the pool at this stage. It was lovely to be in the water, but it did start to slow things down. The contractions were even more intense, but became quite widely spaced apart, giving me enough time to gather strength and be fed bananas by Bob. I was even joking about that being evidence that I was 'letting my monkey do it' (as per Ina May's advice*). There is a picture Bob took of me in the pool with a dreamy smile, something I treasure as a memory of a really positive birth experience! However, adrenaline started to flow again because I got the sense that Eleanor was under a lot of pressure to move things along. She came back into the room after conferring with the Head of Midwifery and said that she needed to see how much further the baby's head had come down since the last contraction because they were slowing up. Something in me knew that I had to do something different to pick up the pace, as I was now being monitored and timed. Every time the baby's heartbeat was checked after a contraction she was fine, so I knew that we were

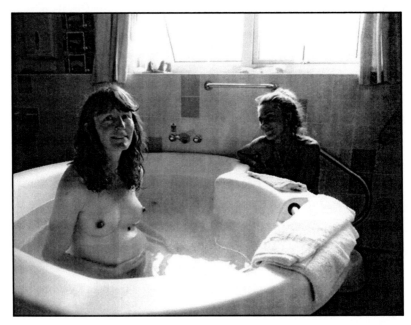

doing well as a pair and I was absolutely determined to avoid any interventions.

I stood up out of the pool with my feet still in the water, but with one leg up on a step and holding on to a bar. I started to do lunges as we had practised during yoga classes and circling my hips like a belly dancer. At one point I put my hand out in a proud gesture, genuinely feeling that I was a 'birth warrior'. Things started to progress and the contractions came with even greater power. I found it harder during this stage for some reason. It was not easy to let the wave of each contraction sweep through me without holding on. I started to understand the importance of really letting go, both physically and emotionally. As well as standing up, I tried squatting right down in the pool, still circling while hanging on to another bar. To cope with each contraction, I was using a mixture of breathing through loose lips like a horse (another technique from Ina May) and loud low groans and roars, all very much from the animal part of me! Jady was also encouraging me to use each breath to push hard down into my bottom. Eleanor stayed a little over her shift to be there at the birth.

Finally, and I don't really remember why or how, I stood up out of the water unsupported and put my hand down to feel my baby's head very low down. She was coming. I had one more contraction and managed to stay standing as the burning sensation told me she was crowning. After having taken her time to get to this point, she came out very fast and took everyone by surprise. Eleanor and Jady had to catch her before she fell into the water! I sat down in the pool with her briefly, but it was very slippery and I had lost a lot of blood, so I had to get out.

I'm not sure how long the second stage of labour lasted but it was around three hours from arrival at the hospital to Clemency's birth just before 8pm, so it was quite lengthy, and the labour ward was busy, so that's why there was a pressure to get me out of the room. Thinking about it in retrospect, it makes me very angry that despite having taken up very little NHS time and resources, by staying at home as long as possible, having a natural birth with no pain relief, and not even staying overnight, there was still a real sense of being hurried up...

Unfortunately, the next midwife on duty had a very different approach to Eleanor, and had a more traditional 'we know best' attitude. I wanted a physiological third stage, but after about an hour she put us under pressure to have the injection. As all of the cord blood had gone to the baby and I was tired and did not want confrontation to spoil the mood, I agreed to this, but

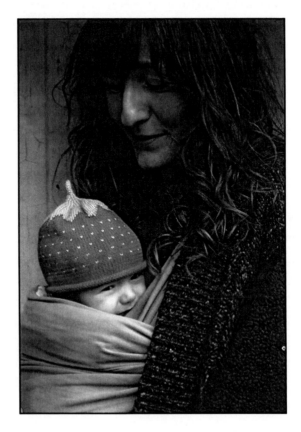

it made me think afterwards how different the birth could have been if we had been unlucky enough to have such an unsympathetic midwife present at the start. The energy in the room was completely different. She was very efficient at stitching me up as I had a tear from the rapid delivery, but lacked any kind of warmth or empathy. But because we insisted on at least waiting an hour for the placenta to come naturally, it meant that we had time together in the room, and Bob and Jady held Clemmie once the cord had been cut. We even had tea and a bit of toast.

Eventually I went to have a shower, as much as anything to have some time to reflect as well as to clean up. I felt incredibly grateful and overwhelmed by the safe birth of my healthy little daughter. I finally accepted the offer of a wheelchair ride to the postnatal ward, and I remember holding Clemmie close and telling her it is a good world to be born into. I was going to stay the night as it was late by now, but Jady offered to stay with us over night at home, and that gave me the confidence to leave the hospital. I really didn't want to be there longer than I had to. We crept out after all the checks telling us our baby was fine, and drove through the night to reach home and begin a new journey as parents.

*Making the decision to have a child — it is momentous. It is to decide forever to have your heart go walking around outside your body.*

**Elizabeth Stone**

# Kristi Keen

*Kristi Keen gave birth to her first daughter three years ago, having an unmedicated, midwife-attended hospital birth. That first experience with natural childbirth was so transformational that it inspired her to become a doula. Here she tells the story of her second birth, so fast that her birth pool stood empty while she took to the shower instead. Kristi is also a professional flautist and resides in Houston, Texas with her husband and two daughters.*

## Kristi's Story

Around 5pm on my 'guess date', I started to notice signs that my waters were leaking. I was not sure, so I just went about my evening as usual. After my husband came home I shared my confusion with him. It seemed like every time I moved, something would leak. We went to bed, and around 3am I woke up to take a usual middle of the night bathroom trip. I saw what I thought was unmistakably amniotic fluid with a tiny bit of blood. I thought maybe I would see my bloody show soon. I had been on the look-out for that for weeks. I decided to try to go back to sleep and hopefully wake up with contractions.

Needless to say I couldn't sleep. Around 4am I woke Robbie up and asked him to keep me company for a while and also asked that he stay home. I texted my midwife and doula just to give them a heads up. I started getting restless and thinking of all the things I needed to do. I asked Robbie if I should blow up the birth pool and he said, 'No, you'll wake the neighbours'. I put the drop cloth down and spread out the birth pool just to have that part done. After that I went and did the dishes that were still in the sink and tidied up as best I could. There wasn't a lot left to do as I had been working on getting our home ready the past few days. Robbie came into the kitchen around 5am to ask what we should do with Lily, our two-year-old daughter. I said, 'I really don't know. It wasn't supposed to happen this way. I was just supposed to have the baby before she woke up.' For whatever reason we just didn't talk about it anymore. I think we went to go prepare the bed at that point. Around 5.30 Robbie decided to get ready for the day and I said I would listen to a Hypnobabies track to try to get more sleep. They always knocked me out.

During the CD I started to get uncomfortable. I denied that they were contractions because they just weren't measurable. They just made me uncomfortable, but it was enough that I started to cry a little. That was weird. After I finished the CD, I went into my room to blow up the pool. I didn't care about the neighbours. I needed something to do to distract me.

I sat on the floor to blow up the pool and it was so uncomfortable having the floor basically push back against my bottom during a contraction. So I started sitting funny. Robbie came out of the bathroom to find me crying because I was so uncomfortable. I felt stupid because it was just too soon to feel that bad. It felt like I had maybe a minute to rest between each contraction. I wasn't timing them. He tried to get me to vocalise through them and I said, 'I'm not ready. I feel stupid. It's too soon!' Robbie called Sandra, my midwife. She asked if she should come. All I could say was, 'I don't know! I don't know! It's too soon! I don't know!' So we waited. Robbie called Jessica, my doula, and she asked if she should come. I said yes. I remember telling him, 'Tell her I am being very irrational'. I remember at that point I was on my hands and knees rocking back and forth and bonking my head against the side of the birth pool. Once Robbie got off the phone I bonked my head against him a few times. He told me that Jessica said if things were going too fast for me then to get in some water. Sandra wanted us to wait to get in the birth pool until she got there, plus it wasn't ready. I opted for the shower.

Because I knew she lived farther away and I wanted Jessica and Sandra there at the same time, I asked Robbie to have Jessica come. Robbie was baffled. 'You want the doula but not the midwife?' I abandoned my efforts with the birth pool and told Robbie to finish it. I was getting in the shower. I put one of my birth balls in there to sit down and let the water flow over me. I couldn't get comfortable. I started to vocalise. I hated the feeling of having the birth ball push up against my bottom during contractions. It was as if it was trying to push the baby back in when it was trying to come out. But I didn't recognise that. I just thought the 'up feeling' was bad.

After a while I got aggravated with the birth ball. I got on my hands and knees during one contraction and then threw that thing out of the shower. I just sat on the floor of the shower and leaned back a little to relieve myself of the 'up feeling'. It helped a little but not much. I heard Jessica come in and it immediately smelled good. I thought, 'Oh, doula!' I couldn't help but appreciate the essential oils. I thought she was wearing them but she told me she put it on the cloth I had nearby. With her there I became a little more honest and even said, 'I hate this!' She reminded me about the baby and started asking me about pushing sensations and whether or not I felt pressure. I did but I still thought it was too soon. I was so mad about how intense it was so quickly that I would growl during contractions. Sandra came in shortly after Jessica got there. I'm glad Robbie just made the decision to call her again because I forgot about that part. I really started feeling the need to poop during the peaks and started yelling, 'Poo poo!' I still didn't think it was the baby. Sandra asked if she could check me. I didn't want her to because I just knew I was just three centimetres. But I said yes. I was complete and my bag of waters was bulging. That was my first and only check of my pregnancy and labour. They mentioned something about getting out and having me labour on the toilet. I said, 'Oh no! Not toilet contractions! I have heard about toilet contractions!' But I got out anyway. I had to spend one contraction on hands and knees first. I didn't like that either.

So I got out and started laboring on the toilet. Not fun! They told me to just go with the downward motion and to push if I felt like it. So I did. It felt terrible but oh so good at the same time. Sandra asked me to reach down to see if I could feel the baby's head. I tried but didn't really feel anything. I kept pushing and felt burn so I said, 'Burn! Burn!' and they had me pant. I had missed that sensation during my first birth. During one push my bag of waters pretty much exploded. Apparently I asked, 'What was that!!???' and nearly shot off the toilet. It was pretty funny.

So before I knew it I was standing up and Robbie was back in the bathroom helping to support me. I remember Sandra doing something with some sort of tool and later found out the baby's head was out and she was suctioning. There had been a bit of meconium*. I gave one last push and the baby was born. Robbie said, 'He's here!' I still hadn't checked to see if the baby was a boy or girl. We had just assumed the baby was a boy the entire time. I sat back down on the toilet holding the baby and just giggled and breathed. I was shaking pretty badly but happy. I can't remember who said it but someone mentioned looking to see what the baby was. A girl! I just laughed and laughed! And then I think Robbie said, 'Oh. Sounds like Lily is awake now.' I had no idea what time it was but things happened exactly like they were supposed to. I had the baby before Lily woke up.

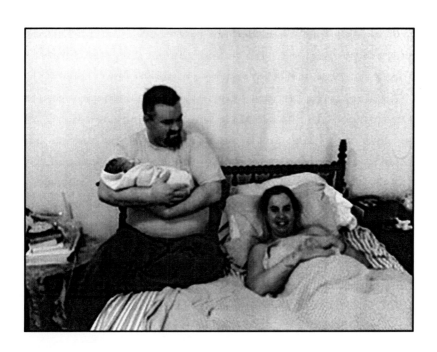

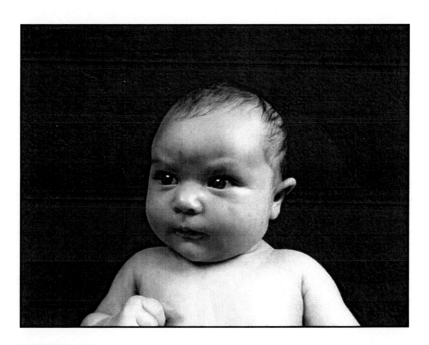

It appears that I laboured for two hours. Nine minutes of that was pushing, but it felt so much longer than that. Kimberly Alexis was born at 8.16am weighing in at 9lbs 4oz.

I told my doula later that I don't think I could have laboured in the birth pool. I said I needed to have living, moving water. With my first birth I laboured in the jacuzzi tub at the hospital and there was something about the bubbles and the whirring of the jets that comforted me. With this birth I needed the movement of the shower. The still birth pool didn't appeal to me at all, even though I thought the entire pregnancy I would want a water birth. I just really like that living water.

# Janet Balaskas

*Janet Balaskas is internationally renowned for pioneering the concept of 'active birth' in the late 1970s. The central concept of active birth — that women should move freely in labour and be led by their body — is underpinned by a deeper philosophy that addresses the dynamics of power in the birth place and calls for women to take an 'active' rather than 'passive' role in their birth experience.*

*Janet is now a leading world voice on birth and maternity practice, and has organised many groundbreaking events including the Water Birth Conference in 1995, pivotal in getting the green light for water births in the NHS by bringing together leading pioneers and researchers from all over the world. She is the founder and director of the Active Birth Centre in London, and the author of several books, including* The Water Birth Book. *Janet lives in London and is the mother of four children, three of whom were born at home.*

*In the story that follows, she tells of the birth of her fourth baby, her first birth using water, at which Michel Odent — renowned water birth pioneer — was her midwife.*

## Janet's Story

I am the mother of four children who were all born naturally and actively. Three were born at home. Although water birth was not yet available, I did enjoy a swim in labour with my third and then carried the memory of the water with me through the rest of my labour.

By the time my son Theo came along it was possible to have a portable birth pool at home. Mine was set up in my bedroom, under the full moon and next to an open fire – so all the elements were there to help me.

The circumstances of this birth were unusual. I was 42, I had had surgery three years before to remove a fibroid leaving me with a scar very similar to a previous caesarean, and he was a very large baby – weighing in at 11lbs or 5 kilos at birth. But as birth is both my profession and my passion, I had some great friends and colleagues on my side for a planned home birth.

Obstetrician Yehudi Gordon was in the background and gave me the go-ahead. And I did live very close to a hospital, so I was not fearful at all and confident I could do it again. My midwife was Michel Odent. I was intrigued by his concept of the 'foetus ejection reflex'* and as this was to be my last baby, I wanted to try it out for myself. This meant that privacy and not too many people around was paramount. I did have my husband at home, but didn't really need him until the very end. I also had a dear friend Mira, who is a midwife, sitting in the kitchen just in case I wanted her. This was reassuring for me as I felt I needed some female energy and did in fact call her to sit with me at some point, although I did not want her to speak or to do anything and apparently told her so in no uncertain terms. Funnily enough, my twelve-year-old daughter was a solace to me. I remember a moment when I looked up out of the birth pool thinking I was going to die and seeing her reading a comic and eating a banana on the bed. So I knew everything was fine as she certainly wasn't looking worried! Soon after this, she was asked to leave the room as Michel insists it is very important that the mother is undisturbed and not feeling observed by anyone as the time of the birth approaches.

He also says that when the word death comes up it means the baby is coming very soon. Sure enough he was whispering to me that it was time to do something different and leave the pool. I later understood that this was because of the anticipated size of the baby and that it was more practical to enlist the help of gravity standing up. I remember following his suggestion, standing up, slowly stepping out of the pool. I tried the all-fours position for a couple of contractions as I had given birth like that the time before, but soon understood I needed to be upright. So I stood up and was supported from behind by my husband. I can't remember much about the timing, but I believe it was about seven minutes later that my son came out in one massive contraction. I remember Michel saying, 'Here is your big boy!' So I had my proof – birth happens most easily and quickly when a woman is undisturbed and free to let go and follow her instincts. It was a perfect 'foetus ejection reflex'. More importantly, it was a perfect birth.

Many elements contributed to this outcome. Not least the support of those around me, their belief that I could do it and their lack of anxiety.

In a practical sense the help of water was immense. This was a very intense and very fast labour. I was very uncomfortable in every position except standing up and bobbing and bending forward. After some time this was getting very tiring and it was such a relief to get into that delicious pool of warm water. Suddenly my body weight (not insignificant with such a big baby) seemed to disappear – I was comfortable in a whole variety of positions. All sense of struggle and strain disappeared. I could relax and let go.

At one moment, soon after getting in, I was squatting and holding onto the edge of the pool, rolling my hips, when I was surprised by an intense orgasmic release.

After that I was in another world where the waves of intensity came and went – I could feel my baby moving down and there were just the two of us doing this – as if we were dancing together in the galaxies. I knew he was coming. I think Michel was wondering about my progress and tried to suggest he might examine me, but I couldn't possibly let him. I thought I heard him mutter something about this being like driving a Ferrari without brakes, but maybe I'm imagining that. It was then I said I felt I was going to die, which must have come as music to his ears… and then it was time to leave the pool. I remember feeling as if I had only just got in – but in fact I was in the pool for about three hours.

In retrospect I can see the wisdom of 'managing' my birth like this – how being in the buoyancy of the water throughout the active phase of labour protected the uterus and optimised the labour, while gravity helped me to have a fast and easy birth.

Michel had just the right blend of respect for my wishes and expert know-how. I'm ever grateful to him for coming with me on this Ferrari ride and 'catching' my beautiful boy.

# Charlotte Dahl

*Charlotte Dahl is a full-time mother to three, wife to one, part-time brand consultant, breastfeeding peer supporter and tennis player. Here she describes her blissful second attempt at water birth in a UK birth centre.*

## Charlotte's Story

Cathartic, empowering, transforming: this is my waterbirth.

The birth of our middle child was incredible. An event I have returned to in my head many times, reliving each moment in detail. Here it is.

I love water. Its calmness and weightless warmth. It seemed the most natural thing in the world to me to want to labour and deliver my babies in water.

2006 was an unusually hot summer. It certainly felt that way to me. I was overdue with our second child, running (or rather lumbering) after my toddler daughter Mimi, grateful for the Wimbledon fortnight (which for once wasn't all delayed by the rain), and willing my body to start labour before 42 weeks which would allow* me the birth centre and water birth experience I so desired.

I had laboured at my local birth centre with our first daughter two years previously and had been so close to delivering in the pool, but due to meconium* in my waters I was transferred at 9cm dilated to hospital. So near yet so far; an operating theatre was the venue for the ventouse delivery that became my reality, shattering my dream of a natural water birth. A beautiful healthy girl made up for the disappointment, but when I fell pregnant again, I was even more determined to give birth in the water.

Fast-forward to 9.30pm on a balmy 5 July 2006. I had just finished my nightly bath and was hauling my 41+3 self out when I felt my first contraction. Cue an excited text to my best friend (a fellow natural birther – she gave birth to twins at home, but that's another story!) then a call to my mum (my other fabulous birthing partner along with my husband.) 'It's begun!'

It didn't take long for labour to establish and I laboured in the garden for an hour or so, playing bat and ball with my husband between contractions (that's active labour for you!). Pressure began to build and I felt I would be meeting our second child soon.

Parents arrive, a race to the birthing centre begins, husband and I in one car, Mum in another (Dad staying at home with the blissfully unaware sleeping Mimi).

At the birthing centre I stride towards the pool, shedding my cotton dress and knickers as I approach, desperate for its warm relief. I love how utterly instinctive natural labour is; you lose all inhibitions, twenty-first-century protocol means nothing. The room was dark and serene, the pool large and inviting. In I get and immediately assume my favourite labouring position, on my knees, leaning forward to ride the contraction, lying back in the pool to recover. In my mind, it's like running on the treadmill or rallying in tennis; you get into a rhythm, focus on your breathing, relax, and tell yourself it's all good. Count the seconds, watch the clock. You can do it. Mind over matter.

The water feels amazing, the weightlessness immediately easing the pressure, making me feel relaxed and in control. Yes it hurts, but it's manageable. The water – somehow taking away the rawness.

The midwife felt no need to examine me. She must have known I was close to delivering.

12am, I ask for gas and air and enjoy the sensation of separating my head from my body. Suddenly the sensation of the contraction changes, and I have an instinctive, unstoppable desire to push, to get my legs as far apart as possible and push push push. My wonderful midwife who has let me labour undisrupted asks me to put down the gas and air to focus on the delivery. I have a moment of comedy madness during the transition phase when I suddenly become aware of the music not being the one special CD I had selected. I manage to roar to my poor husband to, 'Sort the f***ing music out!' Cue husband matching Usain Bolt over 10 seconds as he rushes to change the CD. Then in just a couple of minutes my baby's head is born. One more contraction and all 9lb 3oz of my child is here. The midwife pushes the baby through my legs and I am there, cradling my child, opening perfect legs and announcing to the utter delight of everyone that 'It's a boy'. He is pink and clean with a rosebud mouth and delicate hands. He is the most breathtakingly beautiful boy I have ever seen. Love crashes over me like a wave. The midwife tells us that he was born intact in his sac, my waters only breaking as his body entered the water. So special, so precious, my love.

I climb out of the pool unaided and get on the bed to deliver the placenta. My alert darling boy seeks out my nipple and latches on immediately (a position he maintained for the next 20 months of his life!). We lie together for a while, our senses heightened by the presence of the other.

Placenta delivered, I am ravenous and tuck into the obligatory NHS buttered toast and tea. It tastes like heaven. I am so happy.

My husband takes his child for the first time and cradles him close. He whispers 'my son'. He studies him for a while in the still of the night, trying to work out who he is (we had a shortlist of names, I chose our daughter's so he got to choose our son's). Then he announces, 'Thomas Gabriel, that's who you are'. Our angel boy.

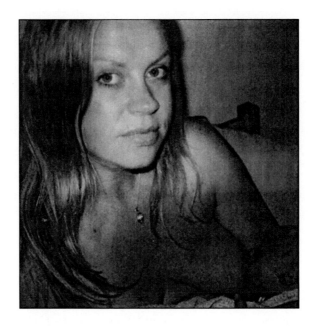

My serene baby snuggles back to my breast and after a while we go to our room. I am feeling good but need to sleep. I quietly congratulate my body for his midnight arrival, meaning we get to sleep in darkness. My husband and mother kiss us both and go, leaving us together, his head on my breast, lulled into sleep by my heartbeat, his comfort for the past nine months.

# Maddie McMahon

*Maddie McMahon is a birth and postnatal doula and childbirth educator. She runs a doula preparation course and combines this with her role as Breastfeeding Counsellor and Tutor with the ABM. Here she describes attending a water birth as a doula, with an unexpected twist. Maddie lives in Cambridge with her husband, one teenage son and a tweenage daughter.*

## A water birth with a difference

'Just pop her in the pool, I'll be there in a while', said the midwife. I took the phone and walked out of the kitchen down the hallway towards the front door. Something was telling me that I'd prefer Jenny to be there before my client got in the water. I knew Jenny well and trusted her implicitly; she was a midwife of the old school, caring, intuitive and passionate about providing holistic care, but something just didn't feel quite right.

'She's really cracking on', I replied. 'I think I'd prefer you to be here before she gets in… I don't fancy catching a baby – that's your job!'

Jenny laughed, told me she'd be twenty minutes and I went back to the birth party. The mother was enjoying her labour. With her partner not around and two of us doulas with her, it was a very female space. We laughed, drank tea, filled the pool and breathed and danced with her through the surges.

It was not before time that Jenny knocked quietly, pushing open the door I'd left on the latch for her and whisperingly announcing her arrival. 'Thank goodness', breathed the mother, grabbing the moment between surges to strip naked and jump in the now-full pool, sighing with relief.

There was a brief time of less-frequent surges. These are the moments when time seems to stop, the world ceases turning and the mother turns inward, resting. Three women sat around the pool in the kitchen, sun streaming through the patio doors, holding the space. 'Hubble, bubble', I thought and smiled to myself.

Almost imperceptibly, the mother was beginning to bear down. It felt so incredibly special to be here with her again – I had supported her through birthing her first child right here, in this kitchen, in this pool.

Up on her knees, leaning over the side of the pool, she was now experiencing the overwhelming expulsive urges that bring the baby down and out. Remembering how she had pushed out her first child, I noticed how her demeanor was different this time. 'What's happening?' she shouted 'It feels different!' All three witches made soothing noises, reminding her to just let her body do the work. Jenny reassured her that all was well. Soon we saw her bottom cheeks open and then her vulva begin to part. 'Please, help!' the mother shouted. 'Something is wrong!' We put our hands on her, looked in her eyes, smiled. 'Let her be born'.

Standing behind her, Jenny and I looked. We saw the slowly advancing 'presenting part' inside the bubble of the still-intact waters. I murmured to my client that she was feeling the waters bulging and that's why it felt odd. As she pushed again, the waters bulged out of her further and further. It looked like she was birthing a huge, mother-of-pearl egg, shimmering under the water.

Slowly the baby advanced into the 'egg' and Jenny and I peered through the membranes, looked at each other and said,

'That baby has a mohican'. We grinned. We looked again. We frowned and looked at each other again and mouthed silently, simultaneously, 'Bum crack!'

There was no going back from here. She was birthing an undiagnosed breech. At home. In water. Not usually a praying doula, I sent a message of thanks upwards that we had Jenny. I knew enough to know that many midwives would at this point be calling 999, telling the mother to get out of the pool and generally causing lots of adrenaline to fly about. Jenny, however, calmly told her that baby was coming bum-first but that it didn't matter, she was just going to birth her baby, just as she did last time.

We fetched the father to come see the baby born and we watched in awe as the bottom advanced, 'rumping' (as they call it – a breech baby can't 'crown'!) and then one leg and very quickly the other and then the rest of the body and head in one swift rush. Calmly, Jenny reached down into the water and gently guided the baby between the mother's legs. Catching her breath, still in the in-between moments of birthing and no-longer-birthing, the mother scooped up her daughter and brought her to the surface.

It was a birth. No big deal. Another wonderful mother birthing in water. I had seen many. But at the same time, how special. What an honour to witness a birth like this. Something I may never see again. I will always be grateful to that mother for inviting me to share her birthing space. She told me afterwards she was so pleased she didn't know the baby was breech. A scan only days before had told her the baby was head down. Her somersaulting baby was blessed; to have an amazing mother and an angel-midwife.

Jenny told me she had thanked her lucky stars that the mother had hopped in the pool as she arrived. Otherwise she might have asked the mother if she could palpate her bump, found the baby to be breech and been bound by protocol to advise transfer to hospital.

Clever somersaulting baby!

# Charlotte Kanyi

*Charlotte Kanyi chose a home water birth with NHS midwives for her first baby. Here she tells of her beautiful, sometimes chaotic, but ultimately life-changing experience. She lives in Birmingham with her husband and two sons and works as a holistic therapist and massage therapist, specialising in supporting women on their journey to motherhood, a path inspired by the birth of her son.*

## Charlotte's Story

I was astonished, but happy, to find myself pregnant a month before we officially started trying. Like many women of our times I knew very little about pregnancy or birth and had little practical experience of looking after babies. I felt excited and terrified in equal measures.

I read widely on the internet and in books to try and fill the vast gaps in my knowledge. Inspired by a couple of friends' births, I already knew I wanted to birth naturally and at home. I learnt more about natural birth through extensive reading, and water birth immediately appealed as I love the water.

A fantasy birth image appeared; a remote woodland next to a log cabin, a roaring fire, me in a hot tub labouring under the stars, listening to the sounds of the night and snowflakes sizzling as they melted on the hot water. However, more pragmatically I was ready to settle for the living room in my home in inner city Birmingham!

My husband was quite taken aback to be asked if he wanted to be at the birth. Well totally flabbergasted is more like it! He is from a rural village in the Gambia where his mother acted as a lay midwife for the women in his compound, none of whom went to the hospital. Birth there is strictly women's business. No men allowed, not even husbands. However, once he got over the astonishment of being asked he was very enthusiastic. He is quite a pioneer, because, as far as he knows, he is the first person in his community to be present at their wife's birth.

I believed strongly in women's innate capability to give birth yet was concerned I might have absorbed some of the fear and misinformation that surrounds childbirth in our culture. Using therapeutic tools, I explored and cleared limiting subconscious beliefs and negative thought patterns that might impede my birth in any way. These included a worry that my birth would be hijacked by the medical establishment interfering. I listened to meditation-style guided visualisation CDs daily, which helped me to grow and maintain my confidence. With my husband we discussed his expectations and fears until he felt relaxed and confident in his supporting role.

With all this in-depth preparation and a month-long trip to the Gambia to get married I was very relaxed as my due date approached. Even though I was likely not to have met the midwives attending my birth and couldn't even guarantee there would be enough on duty, I felt at ease and confident and totally supported. So did my birth pan out as planned? Well… yes and no!

It was Friday and my parents had visited. As they left late in the evening I remarked jokingly that they would be back before they knew it. As I closed the door behind them I felt a twinge that resembled period pains. I wondered if it could be the start of labour then immediately played it down – I didn't want to get my hopes up or look silly if I was wrong. I think I knew really. Still, it was late. I went to bed.

That night felt like one long contraction to me. In reality I was probably mostly asleep, only waking during contractions. Sometimes I barely woke, sometimes I moved onto all fours, gently swaying then lying down to sleep again. As the night progressed they got stronger and closer together. I think they were about every five minutes by the morning. They felt strong. There was some pain but it was different from the kind of pain we have when we have hurt ourselves. It felt 'clean'. I practised taking the label 'pain' off and experiencing the sensations as pure energy and began to appreciate them as signals that I would soon meet my baby and enjoy the labour process. When my husband stroked my back most of the pain disappeared totally as it relaxed me so much and felt so lovely.

When morning came I walked gently round the house relaxing. Well, trying to! I was excited and despite my confidence and preparation some slightly crazy nervous thoughts came up. 'I wonder if that amount of blood is normal or am I haemorrhaging!' for example. I rang the midwives in triage for reassurance and to let them know I was in labour. They were great. They gave helpful practical advice and put me at ease again. I lost the plug* soon after this conversation and my contractions seemed to come more often. I tried to time them for the midwives using an app on my phone but I was hopeless at it. I kept pressing the wrong buttons at the crucial point and wasn't even sure when they were starting and stopping, so I gave up on that and went to see how my husband was faring getting the pool set up.

He was struggling slightly! Pumping had gone well but something was cutting out the hot water and heating (a faulty kettle, we found out later). So he was running up and down the stairs trying to fix that. This wasn't turning out to be the relaxing day cocooned with my husband that I had planned!

Despite the setback with the pool and my unexpected nervous 'crazy thoughts', I remained confident and relaxed. So much so I had some trouble persuading the midwives it was time to come out to me. That I couldn't tell them how long the contractions were didn't help and I was shy to insist, as I had a secret worry that it might only be Braxton Hicks* and I would look silly! At 4.30pm the midwife said, 'It doesn't sound quite time yet, call me again when it hots up a gear'. I put the phone down. It hotted up a gear immediately!

I felt swept up and along by an immense uncontrollable power. Time flew and no longer had any meaning for me and I believe it was 6pm when I rang the midwives again. This time I just said yes to every question and said simply, 'Please come now'.

The community midwife arrived shortly after and was absolutely lovely. Although I didn't know her I immediately liked and connected with her and remained totally relaxed. She was really kind, gentle and respectful, asking me if I had ever had a vaginal exam before and asking permission to do so. I did not know then that it is not always necessary and that I could have said no. Actually in this case it reassured me as she pronounced me 8cm. So I had been right to call them after all! Next question 'Have your waters broken?' 'No'. Whoosh, splat, all over the floor splashing us both. 'Well, they definitely have now,' I said as we both burst out laughing.

I spent some time kneeling by the sofa swaying with my head in the seat. At some point the second midwife arrived. I hesitantly said, 'My body wants to push now'. I was so relieved when my midwife simply said, 'You trust what your body wants to do'. At this stage the pool still wasn't full enough and I was getting worried it would be too late. All I could say was, 'I want to get in the pool now'. They agreed I could labour in it and if it wasn't full as I progressed I could get out for the actual birth. I was so grateful.

Finally stepping over the side and easing myself down into the lovely warm water – at exactly the right temperature according to our thermometer – I felt so joyful. As the water lapped against my body and the warmth penetrated my skin I felt all the tension melt away and with it all pain. I felt no more pain from this time on. As my husband added a couple more buckets and it finally reached the required level I felt totally elated. I had done it – I was in the pool.

I lay back, half floating, half sitting, in a semi-upright position in the pool, my husband stroking my shoulders. My midwife told me my baby's heart rate was good. As I enjoyed the gentle caress of my husband I felt I could drift off to sleep! I was aware of a huge grin on my face the whole time.

My contractions appeared to slow and deepen with longer gaps in between them. I was in the water perhaps an hour and a half in total and had at least ten contractions. I felt there was about half an hour between each contraction, which was impossible. But it felt like that.

In a place of timeless stillness and total relaxation, I surrendered myself to the power of my body and the labour. And it was powerful. I felt the energy rush through me, opening me to the core of my being. I felt as if I was a small droplet of water caught up in the roar of the ocean as it crashed on to the shore after a long journey across continents. I felt the same intensity of power present in an earthquake that causes whole mountain ranges to shudder. I felt exhilarated, joyful and incredibly powerful. It was so simple really. I remained still and my body moved and pushed of its own accord. In between contractions I experienced silence and an exquisite stillness beyond words.

Specific details and timings are hazy during my time in the pool. At some point I asked for the lights to be turned off. I no longer wanted to be touched by my husband as it was distracting me. At another point I was amused to notice my midwives giggling like schoolgirls at the end of the pool, as they tried to see with my head torch. I had one surprising moment when I relaxed even deeper and instead of the usual contraction I experienced my muscles release, and my body simply open and my baby move down slightly. I connected with him and felt him to be calm and relaxed too.

Soon the midwives said, 'Oh – we can see the head – you can touch it'. But I didn't want to. I was enjoying the sensations and feeling exhilarated and didn't want to think about how far or not I had to go. I felt my baby's head pushing to come out and then moving backwards a couple of times. I had a few crazy thoughts come and go that I was taking too long and would be sent to the hospital! I felt some stinging and then suddenly his head was out. Before I had time to reflect, in the same contraction he shot out like a bullet right across the pool! It gave me a really satisfying rush of energy. The midwife gently pushed him back with one finger so that I and my husband could reach him and lift him out together. It was 8.46pm. He rested on my chest serenely, appearing to be asleep, before taking his first breath. I have no words to describe how I felt at this moment and we spent a while just gazing transfixed at his beauty.

I began to feel cold and was helped out of the pool onto the sofa still holding my baby. I held him as my husband counted his toes and fingers for the midwife checks. He licked my nipple but wasn't too interested straight away, opening and closing his eyes a couple of times before appearing to sleep again. At about 9.25pm I felt a contraction and asked to cut the cord, which my husband did after the midwives checked it was no longer pulsing. I stood up and the placenta shot out of me so quickly the poor midwife had no time to catch it and got the second splat of the evening. I felt another surprising rush of satisfaction and joy as it came out. I have since read about the oxytocin that is released on delivery of the placenta and that certainly fits my experience.

Due to our earlier problems with the heating the room was not hot enough really. I had got a little cold and the midwives said baby was too. They were concerned and mentioned hospital if he didn't warm up, so we all got wrapped up in blankets. I made the mistake of not insisting on skin-to-skin and put on his babygro as instructed. Despite this I became a raging furnace to warm my baby. I had read of how the woman's body responds to regulate the baby's temperature and I have to say I have never felt so hot in my life. The midwives were so impressed with the difference in his temperature after only five minutes that they thought they might have made a mistake. I can't know for sure, but I think not. However, I am grateful for this extra incredible experience as it brought home to me again just how amazing we and our bodies are in birth when given the chance.

So the midwives finally left and we remained on the sofa for four hours, cuddling our baby as he suckled, and marvelling in wonder together.

Reflecting back I found the whole birth experience to be fascinating, humbling, opening and extremely empowering. I loved being in the water and once there was able to relax and my confidence soared. This confidence has permeated my life in many subtle ways since. I feel very different and can truly say it was a life-changing experience. I have matured in some way and have a deeper inner confidence and joyful feeling inside. This is something I would like all women to experience, their version of growth and empowerment and joy, and I hope my story contributes to that.

*The moment a child is born, the mother is also born. She never existed before. The woman existed, but the mother, never. A mother is something absolutely new.*

**Osho**

# Emma Lee

*After her plans went out of the window at the birth of her first baby, Emma Lee was determined to feel some control over how she was to deliver again and chose home births. She went on to have three home deliveries, two of them water births, and wishes to share her experiences to inspire confidence, belief and positivity, rather than fear of labour and birth. Emma now has four beautiful children, a husband and is a breastfeeding peer supporter in Nottinghamshire.*

## Emma's Story

*Son one*

I had my first son when I was thirty. I had planned to have a home birth, which was met by opposition from some of my family, mainly because of concern for me and my unborn baby. My mum was unsure and nervous but never said anything to put me off. The concerns were probably due to a lack of knowledge and experience and the fact that home birth isn't the accepted norm. However, I was lucky to have a fantastic midwife in whom I had total and utter confidence, who suggested home birth as an option for me.

I had been in the early stages of labour for twelve hours when the first attending midwife came to our home at about 9pm. Unfortunately, although she was lovely, I think she missed the opportunity to tell me that what I was experiencing was normal and to be expected, to reassure me about what might lie ahead for me, and give me the confidence to stay at home. I had hardly dilated so she left. By midnight the contractions were very painful and felt very frequent, so my husband telephoned the hospital again. Because he was experiencing this all for the first time he was unsure what to say when the hospital asked 'Do you want to come in?' I told him to make a decision, which turned out to be going to hospital! What followed was ok for me as a birthing experience but far from what I felt I wanted or was capable of achieving.

Lots of decisions were made for me but asked as a question, followed by 'Is that OK?' and then carried out anyway, such as breaking my waters, lying me on my back because of monitoring the baby, eating toast (which I threw back up), an episiotomy*, being given gas and air but not told how to use it to work with your contraction so subsequently being totally off my head, and so on. Finally after much distress for all three of us we had a healthy boy at 2.20pm the following day. I found I was out of control of my experience, unable to make the decisions I wanted, frustrated and exhausted! I felt that being on my back for hours on end – incredibly uncomfortable as I had PGP* – contributed to my baby being back to back and then difficult to deliver.

My husband also felt distanced from the experience, as if it were not his own. He felt bored at times, he found it clinical, he felt bewildered by the number of people and midwives we seemed to get through, and ultimately not involved in the delivery of his first child. No two faces seemed to be the same and because the labour was so long our baby was distressed. The room seemed to be flooded with doctors to check on him as soon as he was delivered, which meant lots of other people touched him before me.


*Son two*

Pregnant with my second son I opted for a home birth and was determined to do it.

When the contractions began I immediately phoned my midwife and after a chat she arrived to check on me within a couple of hours. I felt very relaxed and in total control of my emotions, body and decision-making abilities. My midwife was strong, confidence-inspiring and gentle in her manner. She almost whispered what we needed to do next, whether that was to check the baby's heartbeat or move my position slightly. She instilled confidence in me. She encouraged me to move around and ultimately labour and birth on my knees in our lounge as I wanted to. We laughed, talked and focused our efforts together throughout the entire labour.

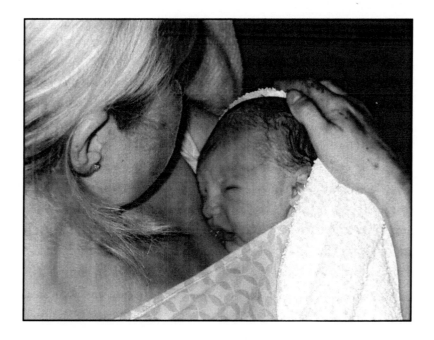

From my previous labour I knew my body was an amazing piece of kit which could do anything. I remember my midwife asking me, 'Can you feel your baby coming down the birth canal?' and I could! At this point I fell in love with my labour and birth.

I held my baby as he entered this world and together my midwife and I rubbed his body to stimulate him and untangle him from his umbilical cord. I had touched him first.

My husband sat on the sofa telephoning our family who could hear the cries of our new baby. He felt like he was completely connected to the delivery of our son; he was free to be involved, make decisions, help and talk to our midwife, ask questions and relax. He didn't find it clinical or stressful and because I was more relaxed he was happy. I was left with just a graze, which felt fantastic compared to the stitches from the episiotomy and exhaustion of a long labour.

### Son three

I had been offered a water birth with son two, which I had turned down because I thought the idea horrible, mainly on the basis that I hate going swimming because it's cold and wet! However, a friend had talked to me about her water birth and how protected and safe she felt, and the idea began to appeal to me. I discussed it with my midwife (the same midwife I'd had previously) and I put into action the process of getting everything ready for a water birth; hosepipe, pool etc. My husband was very supportive and after such a wonderful experience with our second son I think he was happy.

I was warned before the birth that the number of babies due at the same time as us was quite high in our area and that, as a few had opted for home delivery, I might have to go to hospital. This filled me with dread and panic about being bossed about, not free to choose how I wanted to birth in someone else's space and only being able to get into a pool should it be available. My PGP had been especially bad in this pregnancy and I had been told by the physiotherapist not to birth on my back at all.

I struggled to walk most of the time and lying down was quite a challenge!

Anyway labour began, my midwife arrived and I progressed through my labour actively walking around and on a ball. My eldest son, who was three and a half, helped to fill the pool with a cup, which made him feel very important, and when it was full he told me I could go and get my costume on as the pool was ready for me! When I got into the water I felt a calm blanket sweep over me – it was just as my friend had described, only better. I felt comfortable, and both the pelvic pain and the contractions felt more manageable. I could literally feel the rush of happy hormones. The water felt warm, I felt covered, protected and safe and I think what I really enjoyed was the distance it gave me from other people. It hugely increased my personal space and you were allowed in under invitation only!

My greatest concern before labour had been what I should wear in the pool – I'm not a 'get naked' person – but I felt so covered by the water that it felt right for me to remove all of my clothes. In my head I recall feeling that clothes would be in the way of having my baby right next to my skin once born. I remember feeling every bit of the labour and trusting in my body's ability to do its sole purpose in life. I didn't feel I had to work hard to deliver my son, I just let my body do its job, and although very painful, it was a positive pain with each contraction bringing me closer to holding my baby. This labour reaffirmed my love of pregnancy, labour and birthing.

When I felt my baby's head crown I informed my midwife, who was a little surprised, and my husband quickly fetched my mum who was in the garden talking to neighbours and unaware of how imminent the birth was. My fab midwife had turned the lights down low and my husband had put some music on. I delivered to Take That – *The Greatest Day*. As our son was born I turned to take him, with my midwife watching closely next to me, and I held him under the water to visually examine him before I pulled him up into the air and my arms.

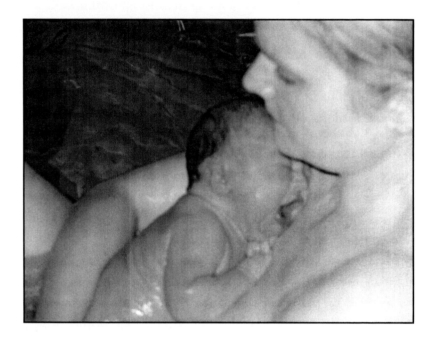

It was one of the most beautiful moments of my life and I was lucky enough to have the opportunity to experience it and share it with people I love. Throughout the labour my midwife, husband, myself and my mum laughed, talked, joked, sat in silence and cried together. I sat in the pool for what seemed like an age after delivery. I could feel the cord pulsating and when it had stopped my husband cut his third son's cord free. The delivery of the placenta was easier in the pool, there was no intervention and it happened naturally with no problems. I was left with a tiny graze and felt invigorated, strong and triumphant as a woman.

*Daughter one (fourth labour)*

No question even needed to be asked of me this time, it was home water birth all the way!!!! My PGP and pelvic problems were severe this time and I struggled to get around, even having to use crutches. I was desperate to deliver my baby and to relieve my pain. I went a day past my due date and unfortunately I was also ill, suffering with bronchitis. The morning of the day I went into labour I was at the doctors collecting a prescription for antibiotics and being told by my very nice doctor that he wanted me to go to hospital should I go into labour. Again the feeling of dread filled my body and panic rose at the thought of what I would do should that actually happen. I immediately said I would speak to my midwife and the doctor said he would speak to her and get back to me.

Off I went home to rest when the first prangs of labour hit me. I waited a while then phoned my midwife, who came round to see me. We worked together at trying to keep me active but I felt so poorly that all I wanted to do was sleep. The pool was ready for action, so she cleared the living room and told me I could have half an hour rest and that then we would deliver our baby. And that is exactly what happened. I slept with contractions for half an hour with my midwife checking on me, and then heard the sound of her voice telling me it was time to get on my feet for the last leg of this labour. It took an hour and one minute from that point for me to get up, dilate 6cm, get in the pool and deliver our baby. Putting it like that it sounds frantic and fast, but it was nothing of the sort – I was about to deliver our baby on my terms and as I wanted.

I was desperate when I got onto my feet to get into the pool, but I needed to be upright to let gravity do its thing and get me to dilate some more. I was on my feet for thirty minutes and then into the pool I slipped. Heavenly. The weight taken off my tummy and pelvis was indescribable, the relief, the comfort and calmness washed over me like a protective blanket as before. Kneeling, I leaned on the side of the pool, which gave me support and the ability to open my knees without feeling like I was splitting my pelvis in half. Again I could feel everything and very quietly I felt my baby's head crowning and the pop of my waters breaking. By myself with my midwife and husband watching I was able to relax and let my body deliver our baby. I took our baby again through my knees and brought her up to my chest and sat in the pool, delivering the placenta naturally.

My husband again said he felt very much part of the support I needed and that he was involved in our family event. Free to move when and where he wanted, eat when he wanted and phone his parents when he wanted. My home and water births are treasured memories and the reasons I want to help other mums and dads to look forward to labour and not fear it. I now work in parent classes and as a breastfeeding peer supporter, and I feel very passionate about promoting normal birth and making women aware of the power that is within them.

# Dianne Garland

*Dianne Garland has been a midwife since 1983 and has been teaching about water birth since 1989. Her work has taken her all over the world, and she has written numerous articles, with a new version of her book* Revisiting Waterbirth – an attitude to care *published by Palgrave in December 2010.*

*Dianne works as an expert witness and university lecturer and maintains her clinical skills on a midwife-led and consultant unit at a local hospital. She is Director for Clinical Governance at Waterbirth International and water birth consultant to Wenzhou Oriental maternity unit in China.*

*Here she shares two different stories of water births she has witnessed: the first, a touching account of empowerment and the rite of passage into motherhood; the second, a tale of how she supported a woman's decision to have her third stage\* in the pool.*

## Amanda's story

I have been supporting women who wish to use water for most of my thirty-year career as a midwife, and just as no two births are the same, neither are two water births. In sharing this birth story I am hoping to give a real feeling of how powerful water can be on several levels. Amanda's birth was a powerful transformation – from single girl, through birth, and into her future life as an empowered mother.

I first met Amanda when I was working in a birth centre she came to look around on one of the regular 'tours'. After we had shown parents around and explained the options for labour and birth within the home-from-home setting, she held back. She was with her mum – no sign of any male companion – and indeed it was her mum who was asking all the questions. Her mum seemed interested in the birthing pool and said that it was just becoming popular when she had had Amanda nineteen years earlier. Amanda remained very quiet and seemed happy to let her mum do all the talking. When they left I gave them direct phone numbers and some other information leaflets about using water and the birth centre facilities.

I was on duty two days later when triage phoned to say that Amanda had come in and was in early labour but wanted to come over to the birth centre. They were keen to send her home but she did not wish to go until she had been assessed (vaginal examination) even though she was only contracting every five minutes. I remembered her and how anxious she had appeared two days earlier and agreed to see her. It is amazing what a familiar face can do. When she saw me she smiled and we actually managed a laugh – at my expense not hers!! I explained that it appeared labour was probably still early and that it was not the best thing to examine her, but would if she insisted. We agreed to let her walk around, go and have something to eat and text her friends to let them know that things seemed to be starting. Three hours later she returned; her waters had gone and she was contracting more strongly, her mum was supporting her physically and emotionally and they appeared very in tune. I examined her and found that she was 4cm dilated and in good labour.

Amanda asked if she could now go in the pool and was a little upset when I told her that the pool would take about forty-five minutes to fill, but that she could go into the shower whilst the pool filled. When a woman goes into water I always say it can take maybe an hour to feel the benefits, as the warm water soothes and relaxes muscles and can enhance the labour. Amanda changed position in the water but after 45 minutes still seemed to be unsettled. I did my usual assessment – lights low, quiet music, water and good room temperature – but somehow the water did not seem to be relaxing Amanda to its full potential.

Whilst chatting to Amanda's mum earlier when Amanda was out of earshot, her mum explained that the father of the baby was not on the scene. He had vanished as soon as Amanda had found out she was pregnant and did not appear to want any input with Amanda or the baby, so her mum had become sole provider – socially, emotionally and financially. This, she said, had put a lot of strain on their relationship.

So back to Amanda in the pool. As I said, she really was not settling and eventually I asked her if there was anything else I could do to make the water more relaxing. Out of the blue she said, 'Could my mum get in the water?'!! Of course the answer was yes. I know some colleagues who find it strange that a birth companion would want to get in the water, so what would they have thought of a mum?! But at the end of the day, it is her labour, choice and decision – not mine. Before I had even had a chance to answer Amanda's question mum was getting her jumper off. I suggested that she might like to wear some theatre scrubs as she had not thought about getting in the pool, so had nothing appropriate to wear. My colleagues duly obliged and brought a pair over from labour ward.

I can only say that the whole atmosphere changed once her mum got in the water. Amanda relaxed, seemed more soothed and changed position, lying in her mum's arms that were doing a great job keeping her calm. As labour progressed they whispered together, words of encouragement and personal support. Within two hours it was obvious that Amanda was getting near to birthing. She changed position, kneeling with her back towards her mum. I explained that the baby would need to be gently nudged forward between Amanda's legs so she could lift her baby out of the water. At the appropriate time I encouraged mum to nudge baby forward into the waiting hands of Amanda. As she bought the baby to the surface she shouted out 'It's a girl!' Up to that point we had not had any conversation about whether they knew the sex of the baby. Amanda was crying, her mum cried and I must admit the emotion got to me as well. Her mum just kept saying, 'I was the first person to touch my grand-daughter'; it was an empowering moment for us all.

After all the usual weighing, measuring and Facebook texts (her generation not mine – I will never understand young people's fascination with social media), we eventually got around to naming the baby. Amanda announced that she would like to call the baby Helen, her mum's name. It was a very emotional moment. The transformation from daughter to mother, and mother to grandmother, was complete.

As a midwife who has assisted mothers with their birth choices for over thirty years, Amanda's birth is still something I will remember for many years to come.

## Mary's story

Mary was having her second baby and had planned to use water this time and hired a pool for use at home. She had only been able to have her labour in water last time as she was booked into a hospital which did not support birth in water. This time she was sure that all being well she wanted to labour, birth and deliver her placenta underwater. It was this last element that got me involved. I was already using water and had delivered third stages underwater without any problems for several years, but Mary's community midwife (Lisa) had never undertaken this and wanted some advice and support. I met with Lisa in our office at the hospital and shared my experiences, the evidence to support the safety of third stage underwater and maybe even more importantly, what issues might alter that plan even during labour or birth.

The most important aspect was to ensure Mary herself was happy with this plan. That was our discussion during our next meeting with Mary at her home; her partner was present and we discussed her plans and expectations, and she shared her disappointment with her last birth when she was asked to leave the water before her son Ryan was born. Mary explained that she did understand why she had had to leave the pool, as the hospital had informed all mothers that they did not have enough midwives trained to support an underwater delivery. What she did not ask was what they were doing to train more midwives!

So with this background we planned Mary's birth at home, which out of interest was an old converted Victorian school house and had the most amazing features – this was surely going to be a beautiful environment within which to birth. Mary had planned for her mum to come over to look after Ryan when she started labour, her pool had arrived (she was now 37 weeks) and they had already set it up in the lounge.

We talked through about being careful about filling it when Ryan was around and ensuring that all efforts were taken to prevent him from getting near the pool unsupervised. I do believe that children can be very resilient and cope well if prepared beforehand when their mum goes into labour. Mary's mum was a little hesitant about both a home and water birth, neither of which choices she could really understand, but after several conversations she understood our role as community midwives and that we were here to provide both continuous professional support and to act as advocates for choice.

When Mary went into labour it was 4am on a cold and damp February morning – not my best time of the day – but when I arrived I found the house ready. Fairy lights set up around the room, an open fire warming the baby clothes, and a very relaxed Mary wandering around making tea and crumpets. If you had not known that she was in labour, you could have been forgiven for thinking that it was just a social event.

About an hour after Lisa and I arrived, Mary said she felt ready to get into the water. Her contractions were every three minutes and on palpation of the baby, all was progressing well. As experienced midwives we did not need to examine Mary vaginally as we all have belief in the woman's own interpretation and knowledge of normal labour and birth. The water washed over Mary's abdomen and she relaxed almost immediately; she hummed and I soon realised that she was gently humming to her baby. I now believe that as midwives our role is to protect both the actual and perceived birth space, so Lisa and I sat quietly by the pool side, her mum busied herself in the kitchen, while Paul her husband sat and kept saying he felt redundant.

And so things continued for about another hour – Mary was humming, barely moving in the water and in the house not even a mouse stirred.

Suddenly we became aware that Mary's humming had changed tone and she was slowly moving in the pool to a squatting position. She gave one small nudge and out came baby Alex, still in his membranes.

Gently she lifted him up and the membrane bag burst, he looked up at her, blinked and was cuddled skin-to-skin in this beautiful gentle environment. We had no time for photographs and did not even get time to call in her mum.

The placenta birthed completely attached within seven minutes, with no bleeding or problems, and they remained in the water for a further twenty-five minutes. We then helped Mary and her new baby out of the pool and she lay down on a settee until baby Alex finished breastfeeding.

It was now about 7am and dawn was just breaking – a bright morning with sun shining over the garden fence in a rural Kentish village which had just added a beautiful element to a beautiful birth. Just as we were all admiring this peaceful environment, Ryan woke up and came charging into the room in his Ninja Turtle pyjamas, shouting to see his new baby. Needless to say, it was not quiet again for some time – but that's birth and especially home water birth: a changing environment which truly reflects the family.

*Remember this, for it is as true as true gets:*
*Your body is not a lemon. You are not a*
*machine. The Creator is not a careless mechanic.*
*Human female bodies have the same potential*
*to give birth well as aardvarks, lions, rhinoceri,*
*elephants, moose, and water buffalo. Even if*
*it has not been your habit throughout your life*
*so far, I recommend that you learn to think*
*positively about your body.*

**Ina May Gaskin**

# Helen Sargeant

*Helen Sargeant is a mother of two boys, an artist and academic who makes work about the female body and her experiences of pregnancy, birth and mothering. In 2012, she formed an arts collective called Mewe comprising visual artists, academics, writers, performers, poets and film-makers who share an interest in and create work about the maternal. Here she shares her water birth story via both poetry and visual art.*

## About my art

**Naoise Birth** is a poem about the birth of my second son. It was a long, slow, and very painful labour, that was physically and mentally difficult. I had a very large fibroid that had grown to the size of a melon during my pregnancy and this posed a very real threat of haemorrhaging. The fear that I felt I believe contributed to the lengthy labour. The most positive experience of my birth, other than meeting my son for the first time, was spending time labouring in the birthing pool. I wished that I had been able to give birth in the water, but due to the haemorrhaging risks had to give birth on land. Naoise was born at the Calderdale Birth Centre, at the Calderdale Royal Hospital in Halifax in 2009.

**Water, Milk** are a series of drawings that aim to capture ideas related to the birth of Naoise. The drawings have been made using pen, ink, pencil and paint. Blown marks expand, burst and pop onto the surface of the paper. While making these marks I was thinking about eggs, fertilisation, control, and lack of control in the conception of a child. About blowing soap bubbles through my hands to entertain my children at bath time.

Elemental colours have been used, blue for water, red for blood, the white of the paper for the body and flesh of the birthing woman. The amorphous body depicted reaches to the very perimeters of the paper, breasts and nipples touch the edges to convey ideas of the body seeping into the water and space of the birthing pool, the flesh of the body and water becoming one. Circular graphical motifs feature throughout to symbolise the passing of time and represent life cycles. Lines and arrows are used to create tension within the work and relate to painful contractions felt in labour.

## Naoise Birth

The last milk pearls glisten on my nipples
Your first movements began as a tickle
A minnow swimming
Safe
A melon sized fibroid had grown in my womb
Crowding your room
It threatened to cause me to haemorrhage during birth
Blood rivers flooded my mind
Fear
Water slowly filled the pool
Contractions squeezed hard
I clambered on a stool as if mountain
My body became submerged
Comfort
Holding
Hugging
Caressing
Soothing
Water

Circling, floating, twisting and turning
A dolphin
The first woman born
You inside your amniotic fluid sack
A Russian doll swimming pool
Happy
I am the porch, the threshold of the universe
Your birth on land was long
Time in the water
Holds heavenly memories of
Love
Meeting you holding you, seeing your ice blue eyes
Feeling your soft peachy skin
Looking at your downy hair
Feeding you from my breast
Is the moment of birth without language?
the woman is open
she speaks with cervix
she speaks with her voice
that is her body
one body separating
the self, the other
mother, child

# Milk, Water I

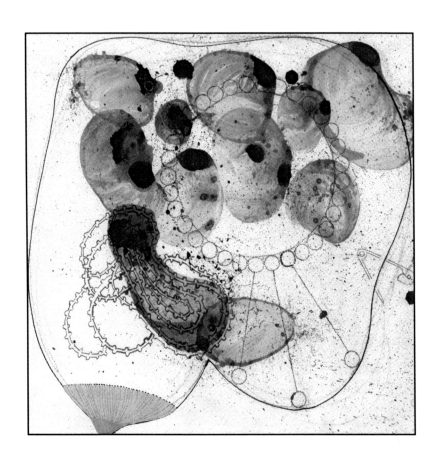

# Milk, Water II

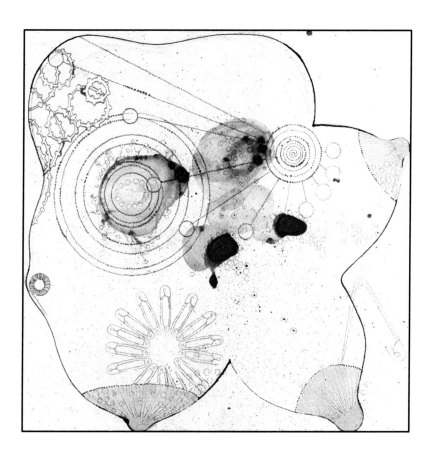

# Milk, Water III

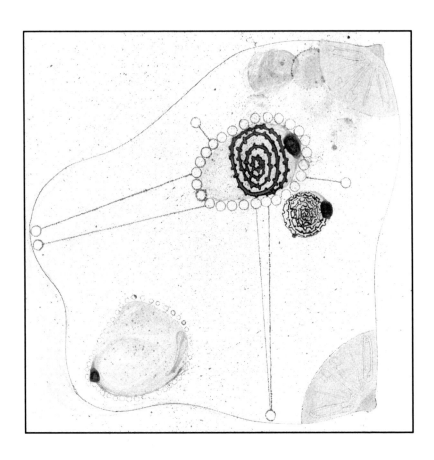

# Pria Holmes

*Pria Holmes lives in Melbourne, Australia with her husband and son Caspar. Her story describes her first birth at home in water, an experience so positive it has inspired her to train as a midwife. She also hopes to birth many more babies at home.*

## Pria's Story

After being frustrated for weeks that I had been waking each morning without you in my arms, I decided I needed to let go and trust that you would come when you were ready. I was 41 weeks and five days pregnant and your dad and I climbed into bed just before midnight. Just as I surrendered to sleep, I was woken by huge surge of pressure. It subsided quickly so I checked the time – 12.15am – and wriggled back under the covers.

It happened again. Now it was 12.23am.

Ah! Unmistakable. Labour! Finally!

Your dad stirred. I told him you were on your way and to keep sleeping. I knew it was early and I needed to conserve my energy. I fell asleep with my hand on my belly and woke every eight minutes throughout the night.

I rose with the sun and dozed on the couch in between surges. When I couldn't sleep any more, I talked to you about what lay ahead. I sent a text to our midwife G at 11.31am to let her know we would need her in the coming hours. Her reply, 'Lovely, stay in touch. Talk soon x' filled me with confidence.

By then surges were six minutes apart and had been happening regularly for just over twelve hours. I sat on a birth ball and focused inwards, circling my hips and singing to you through each surge. I say surges and not contractions because that's what they were – surges of warmth and energy that took me deeper into myself. Each one expanded my heart and body and left me feeling hazy. Like afterglow.

Your dad and I shared our last meal together and set up a pillow mountain for me to drape myself over. We tried to watch a movie but had to stop every five minutes so I could rock on all fours while your Dad massaged my sacrum. It approached midnight and I sent him to bed. I smiled in the quiet darkness, loving feeling us work together. I rested my hands on my stomach and thanked you for teaching me to appreciate my body. I told you I would miss feeling you move in my belly and you kicked my hands. Surges became stronger and closer together after that moment.

I started vocalising through them and was keeping my head down and eyes closed, trance-like. Your dad returned to me after only a couple of hours of sleep – today was his birthday! I was starting to feel exhausted and asked your dad to call G. She arrived just after 3am and sat with me through a few surges, encouraging me to make low sounds. G said we were doing wonderfully and sent us to bed. I managed to sleep in between surges for a few hours and woke after another sunrise feeling well rested.

I had a long shower, savouring the hot water. G told me she could tell from my voice that we were making good progress. I kept moving and when my belly tightened and released, I closed my eyes, breathed and moaned. The surges were longer and closer together, their centre much deeper in my pelvis than before. Your body had noticeably descended. After listening to your perfect little heartbeat I asked your dad to prepare the pool. I stayed in our bedroom working through surges with G at my side reminding me to relax my shoulders and relax my jaw.

I was starting to feel fatigued when your dad came to say the pool was ready. I waddled into the lounge room, undressed and submerged myself in the warm water. I floated on my back, finally weightless and able to rest my swollen body. Each time a surge started to wash over me I flipped over and my attendants poured water over my back. After each one, I rested my head on the edge of the pool and slept until the next one roused me. It was blissful and easy. Your weary Dad asked G if she thought we'd see our baby today. She smiled and said, 'Wouldn't that be nice!'

I spent hours in the pool and eventually needed to get out to go to the bathroom. Giggling at my prune-like waterlogged fingers was cut short when the intensity of a surge doubled me over and left me breathless. I could feel my shoulders and thighs tense as I felt a surge beginning, bracing myself. For the first time I felt pain rather than energy, pressure and intensity.

G suggested spending some time on land to create some more space in my pelvis. I did sideways lunges with one foot up on the stairs. I was scared of the pain and seized up, trying to escape it. My legs shook and I whimpered and complained. G reminded me that this work was making room for you to move down and to not be afraid. She massaged my thighs and soothed me with reassuring words. I found my groove again and started to enjoy feeling my body being so productive. I was surprised by my strength and the more I relaxed into it, the less pain I felt.

When my legs started to falter under my weight, I returned to the pool and promptly vomited over the side. Surges were much more intense and despite the weightlessness I struggled to get comfortable. G called the second midwife, M, who arrived while I was working through a formidable surge. I could feel her presence in the room and looked up to see her, wide-eyed and smiling as she watched me.

I climbed out of the pool again, hot and uncomfortable. The pressure on my cervix was immense and it was difficult to walk. I felt stuck and started to doubt whether I could labour for much longer. I decided to ask G to check my cervix. She and your dad reassured me that we were progressing wonderfully and that you would be born regardless of an exam. I considered it for a few minutes and insisted that I did want G to check. She was so gentle but having to lie on my back, even for a few moments, was unbearable. G told me that my cervix was fully dilated on one side and 7cm on the other – you hadn't fully rotated your body just yet. She told me that to help you the most useful thing to do would be to lie on my left side with my right leg slung across my body and to stay there for about 40 minutes. She warned me that it would be difficult. It seemed impossible.

I tried to get comfortable but a surge began and as it peaked, I screamed. Lying still when I desperately needed to get up and move felt so counterintuitive. I shouted that I couldn't do it. Your dad held me tight and G massaged my feet and ankles and it was soon over. After struggling through a few surges I found a rhythm and all of us slept in between each one. It felt like fifteen minutes later when I needed to go to the bathroom and was shocked when G told me an hour had passed. The downwards pressure in my pelvis was unbelievable and I waddled quickly to the bathroom, hoping to avoid any surges while I was there. Once I sat down I vomited across the floor and heard an audible pop. Your protective bag of fluid had finally released. I called out to G and M, 'uhh…I think my waters broke.' G shouted back, 'I know! We heard it!' It was 6.47pm on Sunday.

I tried to bounce on the fit ball but felt too unsteady. Surges were coming over the top of each other and I could barely catch my breath between them. I wanted to get back in the pool but the water was cold. M started reheating it and I returned to the bedroom. I was exhausted and started to panic. I cried and told your dad I couldn't do this. I was just a little girl. Not ready to grow up. Not strong enough for this. Not ready for a baby. I said you were never coming. G told me that when I said that, she knew I was very close to meeting you. The logical part of my brain understood that this meant I was transitioning, but I still didn't believe her. I growled that I wanted a caesarean. Your dad told me I was doing beautifully. G told me to trust my body and go with it.

Just surrender. Let go.

I whimpered and insisted again that you were never coming. I asked again for a caesarean. I couldn't do it. Your dad told me I was doing it and that the pool was almost ready for me.

With the promise of the pool, I focused and decided to move forward. It was time to claim this birth and time to be independent. Time to grow up. Time to be a woman.

I called out to you, 'Come on baby!!'

I immediately felt a rush of energy, as though I'd just woken up from a long sleep. Your head dropped through my cervix and started to descend.

'Oh wow the baby's coming! I can feel it moving down.'

I dropped to my hands and knees, hips low to the floor. I roared. Roared like a lioness. Instinct took over and my body involuntarily pushed with each surge. I was primal and animal and LOUD. I could feel your every move and was captivated by how powerful we were. We felt incredible. This was our beginning.

Our awakening.

The pool was finally ready and I got up, power walked to the lounge room and climbed in. I kneeled and reached down to stroke your head, poised to emerge. I felt the next surge build, squeezed your Dad's hands and roared. I heard G remind me to breathe, to slow down. Another surge started and as it peaked, I thought my pelvis would split in half but then immediately came sweet relief. G told me your head was born, that your shoulders were rotating and with the next one, you would be here.

I breathed, waiting for the next rush. One final roar and I felt your slippery body wriggle through mine. I turned over to see you under the water.

You were white, with your eyes closed and arms outstretched with long fingers extended.

I scooped you out of the water and brought you to my chest. I said hello and told you we had been waiting so long for you. You opened your eyes and looked up at me but hadn't yet taken a breath. I kept saying hello as I rubbed your chest and tickled your tiny feet, calling you in. I blew gently on your face and you joined us. You took your first breath and let out a big cry.

Hello baby!

I kissed your dad and told him I wanted to do it again. I asked what day it was. 8.55pm on Sunday 20 November 2011. You share your birthday with your dad! We marvelled at your beautiful dark hair and long toes. Realising we didn't know your sex, I unlooped your cord from around your ankle and moved it aside.

A little boy! Wow! Our baby boy. Welcome Earthside, baby.

We started to get cool in the water so climbed out and sat on the couch. You looked for my breast and attached easily. After about an hour, I felt your placenta separate but I was too interested in you to make any effort to birth it. G helped me wiggle forward on the couch and with one push, it was out. I wanted to shower and get into bed and asked if we could cut your umbilical cord. G explained to you that she was going to clamp your cord and then your dad would cut it. She reassured you that it wouldn't hurt. I will always be grateful that the only person to touch you in the first hours after your birth apart from your dad and I, showed you respect, reverence and love.

I showered while you and your dad cuddled, skin-to-skin. We climbed into bed together and our midwives tucked us in, leaving just after midnight. Your dad and I smiled at each other, kissed you goodnight and we fell asleep together.

Your birth changed me forever; it made me a Mama. It also forced me to see and accept my strength and my vulnerability. I worked hard to birth you. It was blissful, rewarding work. More rewarding than I ever could have imagined. And yet, while life changing and transcendental and blissful, your birth was also perfectly ordinary, normal and uneventful. You were in my arms and it was like you had always been here.

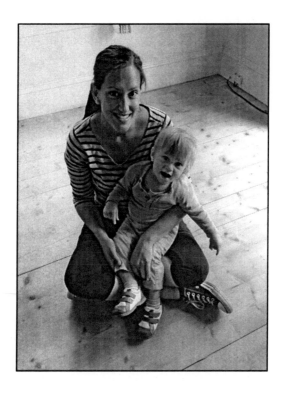

*These things you keep*
*You'd better throw them away*
*You wanna turn your back*
*On your soulless days*
*Once you were tethered*
*And now you are free*
*Once you were tethered*
*Well now you are free*
*That was the river*
*This is the sea!*

**The Waterboys**

# Sarah Banks

*Sarah Banks planned a home water birth with her first baby but had to transfer to hospital. Second time around she achieved her home water birth and it was even more magical than she could have imagined. Sarah lives in Derbyshire with her husband and two daughters.*

## Sarah's Story

Sophie Faith Banks was born in water at home, weighing 8lb 7oz. This is the story of her amazing birth.

I woke at around 3am and felt wet, went to the bathroom and it seemed like my waters had gone. I tried to go back to sleep but was getting contractions on and off and wasn't comfy in bed, so I got up and came downstairs and watched telly whilst sitting on my birth ball. By about 6.30am I felt that the contractions were getting a bit closer so I woke Dave up and asked him to start timing them – they were about twenty minutes apart.

We pottered around with our eldest daughter Molly and had some breakfast. I spent most of my time on the ball as it was the most comfortable place to be.

We rang our doula Stephanie and she arrived at about 10am, by which point I was baking cakes with Molly – she was getting bored as we'd decided to keep her off nursery. I was still having contractions regularly and using the breathing techniques I'd learnt at the Mindful Mamma class to relax through them.

By about noon my contractions were coming every three minutes and I was sat on a chair with Stephanie massaging my back. As they were getting closer and longer Dave started to get the birth pool ready with Molly before taking her over to her friend's house, whilst Stephanie and I had some lunch. Things slowed down a little while I ate but then went back to every three minutes, so, at about 2pm, we decided to call the midwife.

The midwife arrived just after 3pm and I was in the dining room breathing through my contractions whilst Stephanie continued to massage my back. Everything was going well and I was well into my birthing zone. The midwife spoke to Dave and wanted to examine me, so reluctantly I came out of my zone and went into the living room – by this point it was 3.45pm. I was a little disheartened as despite my birth plan clearly stating that I didn't want to be told of my progress she informed me I was 4cm whilst she was still examining me and added that my waters hadn't actually gone. As her shift was due to end at 4pm she said she wouldn't stay, but asked if I could I provide a urine sample before she left.

Dave and I went up to the bathroom – I was feeling quite disheartened after the 'progress report' – and we spent about half an hour up there so that I could re-establish my breathing and get back into my zone – I didn't even try to provide a sample! During this time the new shift of midwives arrived.

After our time in the bathroom I could feel pressure building and said that I felt the baby wouldn't be long – so it seemed that this magic time in the bathroom had helped things progress quickly.

I came back to the dining room and Dave spoke to the midwives, who were very happy to leave me to get on with things. I wasn't really aware of time but I'm told that I only got into the pool at about 5.20pm as both Stephanie and Dave felt I was in transition.

I remember being totally relaxed in the pool, breathing through the contractions and visualising my baby moving down.

Dave was sat at the side of the pool talking to me, and Stephanie asked me if I could feel baby's head – I could, but she was still a few centimetres inside. The midwives came in and checked the pool and Stephanie went to get some more hot water as they said it was too cold.

Whilst Stephanie was in the kitchen I looked down and was amazed to see my baby, floating in the water in front of me! I had obviously breathed her out and she had taken everyone by surprise – even me! I wish we had a video so we could see just what had happened but can only assume that she must have swum up to me.

I lifted her out of the water and was passed my glasses so that Dave and I could see her sex for ourselves. Sophie was a perfectly healthy little girl, covered in vernix. There had been no shouting, no pushing and no drugs.

I left the pool for the third stage and after about half an hour of being fed cake and tea, my placenta was delivered naturally, still attached to Sophie.

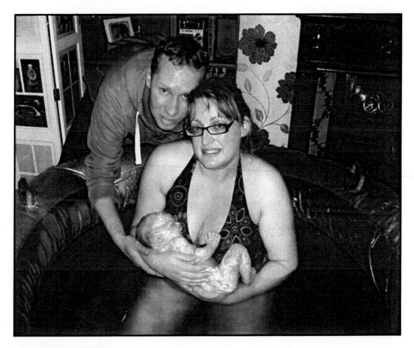

Just over an hour after Sophie's birth I had a lovely bath. Molly came home briefly to meet her new sister before going back to her friends for a sleepover, and by 9pm Dave, Sophie and I were tucked up on the sofa eating egg and chips.

# Lisa Marinou

*Lisa Marinou had her first child by emergency caesarean and her second and third children by elective caesareans. Finally, with baby number four, she had the birth she had always dreamed of – a HWBA3C (Home Water Birth After 3 Caesareans)! Lisa and her husband Panayiotis live in the West Midlands.*

## Lisa's Story

Finally I got my little pink line!

I already had three children but after having an ectopic pregnancy it took us nine months to conceive. My husband and I were thrilled but unfortunately it was a double-edged sword as we knew a battle lay ahead.

My first daughter was born by crash emergency caesarean for what I believed to be some sort of placental abruption. I was never really given any explanation but I guessed it must have been serious. The recovery period from this surgery was not easy and was compounded by postnatal depression, which I believed was a direct result of the trauma surrounding the need for surgery. I had needed a general anaesthetic so knew nothing of my baby being born. When I fell pregnant with my second child, I asked my local hospital to support me in trying for the normal birth I had always wanted but sadly missed out on the first time – but not for want of reading and studying all I could. Unfortunately I was given no support and told if I wanted to be awake to see my child born I would need to have another section, this time elective. I was heartbroken at this news, but wanted to avoid another emergency, and I felt I was not offered any choices and had no real options. My second daughter was born and I was awake which was lovely, but I still felt I was missing out as a woman and a mother, not being able to be given the chance to birth our child.

Soon after this I was pregnant again with my son. Again I approached my local hospital to support me in attempting a vaginal birth after two caesarean sections (VBA2C). The reception this time was worse than ever. Firstly I was told that not only would I need another section, but secondly I would need to be sterilised! I refused sterilisation, only to be met with 'Don't you think three children are enough?' And as for trying for a VBA2C, my consultant told me in no uncertain terms, 'If you want to kill yourself and your baby – that is your choice!' Obviously upon hearing this, another elective caesarean section was booked. I was also told that I had suffered a heavy blood loss at my last birth so was now at increased risk of haemorrhage; the loss had been documented at 700mls. However, what came from these discussions was the fact that this consultant could not find any evidence of a placental abruption in my first birth. I had to ask myself – had I been put through surgery three times for no apparent reason??

So here we were with baby number four. After extensive research, I believed it was a safe option, under close supervision, to attempt a VBA3C (vaginal birth after three caesarean sections). My dream was to be at home and in water but I wondered if this was too much to ask for? I needed to find a health professional with the experience and confidence to support me. I obviously approached my hospital first, but again they showed absolute horror at the mere thought of a vaginal birth after three caesareans – I did not mention the home and water bit! I had to think to myself, was my uterus going to rupture at the mere thought of labour and birth – what exactly were my risks and how did they compare to the surgical risks of a fourth caesarean section? Upon more research I came to meet a doula who herself had achieved a VBA3C and from there came across the work of independent midwives. I was introduced to an Independent Midwife* who had specialised in VBAC after her own experiences of VBAC in hospital. She looked into my previous pregnancies and births and we discussed at great length all aspects of these births to assess what my absolute risk factors were, if there was any chance I could safely attempt a VBA3C and where the most appropriate place to birth was. She found nothing to categorise me as high risk apart from the fact I had had three sections, so we asked her if she would be our midwife and thank God she agreed. My dream had been to birth at home and in water, and although my independent midwife could not guarantee that would happen, she saw no major reason why we could not plan a home water birth – there was evidence to suggest that this was actually a good plan. I had watched a YouTube video of a successful home birth after four caesareans and thought, if that woman can do it – so can I!

Now to put my team together.

My midwife contacted my consultant at the hospital to notify him of our intentions and after making it clear that I was aware of all the risks involved, and that it was my decision to go on this journey, he respectfully agreed to support our decision for a home birth and let us know that if at any time we needed help he would be there. This was of great relief to me, as it meant no more fighting. I could enjoy my pregnancy and prepare myself for the birth. I now actually had to think – 'I am going to give birth normally'.

My pregnancy continued without complications and my due date came and went. I was suddenly at 42 weeks pregnant and so made an appointment to see the consultant at 42+3 to talk about options... I believed my dream might be slipping away. My midwife kept my spirits high and told me to trust in my body as things were happening and going in the right direction. After two nights of false starts, my body went into labour, coincidentally the night before the consultant's appointment!

Once my contractions reached five minutes apart I asked my husband to call my midwife. We have never been so relieved to see someone in all our lives! By this time I was ready to transfer in if there had been no progress – I needed to know.

Upon examination I was found to be 7cms dilated!! And my midwife announced 'Let's cancel the appointment and have your baby at home today'!!! I was thrilled beyond words. There I was in the birthing pool, in my lounge with my husband, two midwives and my doula – my team, people I trusted, in surroundings which were familiar and comfortable. With encouraging words and support I progressed quickly and before I knew it I was bearing down. I always wondered what this would feel like and 'Would I know?' - the answer is yes, I knew, and my body did not need any encouragement – it knew exactly what to do. I gave birth to my daughter myself in the pool and lifted her to my chest, my beautiful baby in my arms, born the way I always dreamed of – totally naturally.

As a woman and mother I now feel complete, and I will be eternally grateful to my Independent Midwife for supporting me and believing in me to make my dream come true. Now I feel totally empowered and can take on the world. VBAC after multiple caesareans does not have to be a process to be managed at every point because of a perceived risk factor that cannot actually be measured correctly. Not enough women are given the choice and the support to attempt it and so there are no detailed statistics available. My midwife contacted my consultant to let him know all went well and he wrote back, 'CONGRATULATIONS and well done'. This was amazing to receive as I had

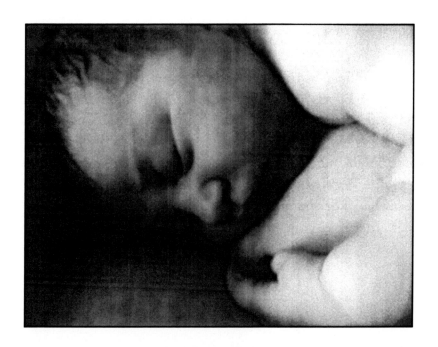

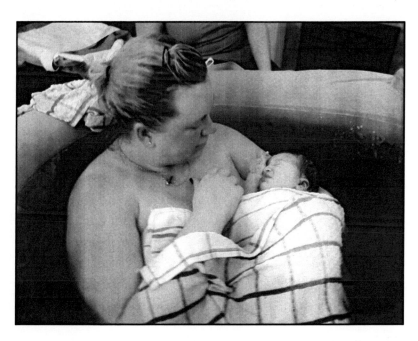

heard lots about responses along the lines of 'You were lucky this time', aimed at VBAC women. My team of two midwives, a doula and consultant obstetrician, working together with my husband and I, with the expertise being utilised in the correct manner and according to clinical need, is how it is supposed to work for all women with perceived risks. It can and does work – I am proof.

# Sarah Ockwell-Smith

*Sarah Ockwell-Smith had her first two babies in hospital after she was transferred in from planned homebirths. Her third and fourth babies were born at home in water, against medical advice due to her history of 'big babies' and high blood pressure. Here she tells of how her third birth and first water birth healed the trauma of her first two births and of the magical effect the water had on her body. Sarah lives in Essex with her husband, four children, three cats and nine chickens and is a parenting author and founder of BabyCalm.*

## Rafferty's water birth

Rafferty is my third child and my first baby to be born in water, at home. I had hoped to have all of my babies this way, but fate had other ideas. My first labour was very long and painful and after three days of pre-labour and ten hours of established labour I was transferred to hospital for augmentation and an epidural. My difficult labour was blamed on my son's weight (10lb), but retrospectively I now know that it was really down to a lack of support and fear. My 'failure to progress' was not really a failure of my body at all – rather I had been failed by 'the system', and my mind was too full of fear from all that society had instilled in me.

Five months later I was pregnant with my second baby and, determined to enjoy the experience this time around, I prepared myself as best I could. I visited a hypnotherapist to try to help me release some of the trauma I had retained from my first birth and I read every positive book I could find. I felt that I was finally well prepared and, although I was nervous, I was looking forward to labour this time. My birthing pool was set up and I had arranged my 'nest' in the room I hoped to birth in. I had high hopes that all would be well. However, a day after my due date I was diagnosed with pre-eclampsia*. My blood pressure had been high with my first baby but never progressed to anything more serious, but this time it was through the roof and my body was leaking protein. I was admitted to hospital, monitored for two days and finally induced.

I was desperate to use the birthing pool, but I was told that as I was 'high risk' this was not possible. My labour started swiftly after one dose of prostin and thankfully I had a very straight-forward delivery – four hours from start to finish. However, because of the stress of the environment I found myself in, I was unable to relax and my adrenaline levels were through the roof. Unsurprisingly I found it hard to cope with the pain and requested an epidural. My 9lb 12oz, screaming son was born covered in meconium twenty minutes after the epidural was sited. I was naturally happy that I had another beautiful son, but his birth, combined with the disappointment of the first, left me feeling flat. Everyone told me that I should 'count myself lucky' that I had two healthy babies and I felt guilty for even thinking negatively about their births. I was told 'that doesn't matter now' – only it did matter to me, and I carried the burden of their births and the disappointment I felt into motherhood with me.

When I found out I was expecting for the third time, despite an awful lot of ridicule and negativity from others, I decided that I needed to have one last try at having a home water birth. In some ways I felt I needed a good experience to prove to myself that I could birth naturally, and I didn't care what anybody else thought, I was doing it only for myself and for my baby.

As expected though, given my previous history of pre-eclampsia* and macrosomia*, I had hurdles from day one. I was classed as high risk because of my previous 'big babies' (9lb 12oz and 10lbs) and the pre-eclampsia I had with my second baby.

It appeared I had been assigned the most anti-home birth consultant at our local hospital. At my first appointment, upon hearing my plans for my birth, he scrawled all over my notes in red pen: 'Homebirth not Advised', telling me that the safest option would be an early induction. He explained that he felt my baby was likely to be 'exceptionally large' and that since I, at 5 feet 1 inch, was not, I would be jeopardising the life of my child by birthing at home. I don't know how I found the strength, but somehow I managed to thank him for his opinion and told him that I was sticking to my plans. I also refused the GTT* that I was told I 'must have', having taken one in my last pregnancy with perfectly normal results. I did consent to one growth scan at 32 weeks, at which I was told that my baby was 'already 7lbs 2oz' and an early induction was strongly recommended once again.

My pregnancy progressed smoothly (well as smoothly as it can when you have two under two to look after!) until my 36-week midwife appointment, when I was told that my baby was lying in a transverse position, and that, due to his size, they strongly suspected that he was too big to turn. One week later, however, after an awful lot of moxibustion* and positioning exercises and much to everyone's surprise, the baby turned head down. Despite the negativity of the hospital staff, my community midwives were really supportive of my plans – that is, until the day before my due date, when my fabulously well-behaved blood pressure went up to 150/110.

I was sent immediately to hospital for imprisonment (sorry, I mean monitoring); it was like a rerun of my second birth. This time though my liver function and urine testing came back clear. It seemed I didn't have pre-eclampsia, 'just' pregnancy-induced hypertension. After a long discussion about the risks of me continuing with my plans I struck a deal with the doctors that I could go home on bed rest and have daily blood pressure checks done by my community midwives. They explained that I could avoid being readmitted as long as my diastolic reading never went over 95. Just before I left they scrawled over my notes 'Still wants a homebirth after being advised of medical risks'.

Two days later, one day after my due date, I lost my mucous plug and the next morning I started having mild contractions sporadically. I had planned to birth with my first two children around me, but my body clearly had other ideas, as my contractions kept petering out every time the boys came near me, and they stopped totally that night. The next day, now 40+3, the same thing happened again. I took myself off for some reflexology that evening, which gave me the best night's sleep I'd had in ages. However, I woke to nothing – none of the niggly contractions I'd had for the previous two days. My husband decided to go into work late so that he could look after the boys and I could have some rest in bed.

By the time the regular morning chat show came on the TV I realised that I'd been contracting roughly five minutes apart and wondered if things might finally be happening. I went downstairs and shut myself away in the study, which I had set up as the birthing room with my pool, lots of candles, beanbags and duvets. It was a chilly day in early January so I drew the curtains, cranked up the central heating, burnt some clary sage essential oil, lit my candles and shut the door on the boys so that I couldn't hear them. The boys had other ideas though and kept coming into the room trying to talk to me and play with me. At this point I realised that I couldn't labour with them around me so we called a friend to take the boys out for the day and phoned for a midwife. The midwife arrived an hour later and, as I was unsure whether or not I was really in labour, I asked her to examine me. The contractions had become irregular again and were very mild in intensity. After a quick examination and lots of reassurance on her behalf the midwife told me she was staying – in reply I told her she'd be in for a long day if she did! At this point I didn't have much faith in my ability to really do this.

I spent the rest of the morning rocking around on my birth ball, watching various dire morning television programmes. My blood pressure began to creep up and was just shy of 95 (our agreed transfer level) so I decided it was time for the pool. My notes say I got in at 3pm. My diastolic blood pressure immediately dropped to 65, lower than my booking reading, and my contractions lessened in intensity. I was immensely grateful for the soothing effect of the water, but was concerned at the thought that this meant everything would slow down or stop completely, as it had in my first labour. Looking back I know it was just because I was so relaxed by the cocoon of the warm water.

We had hired a pool with a heater and filtration unit and I cannot recommend these enough, despite the extra expense. I had used the pool every night for a fortnight before for my hip pains (I had been diagnosed with PGP*) so I felt really at home in it and knew how I was most comfortable. I also added some lavender and neroli oil to the water; again, I had been using these every night and had a strong sense of relaxation conditioned to them. By about 3.30pm my contractions were starting to bite a bit and the midwives had to really help me keep calm and breathe through them. Despite the intensity of my labour I felt in control and never felt any need for pain relief.

In my previous labours my waters had been broken artificially so I had no idea what it was like for them to break spontaneously, but I soon felt a pop and a gush and told the midwife that either my waters had gone or I had just lost all control and had a giant pee in the pool. She smiled and told me she was almost certain that it was my waters, and at this news I felt very proud of myself that for the first time in three births I'd avoided the dreaded amni-hook*.

At around 3.45pm any pain I had been feeling all moved into my lower back and I realised that my body had started to bear down. The midwives asked me if I could examine myself and explain what I felt – I however felt nothing but some pretty grim bulging and a handful of piles! They asked me if I could feel a head and I told them I really had no idea what I could feel, but that there wasn't a head there unless I was giving birth to a giant haemorrhoid. Despite my discovery they clearly thought things were imminent as they donned their fetching plastic aprons and gloves. Upon seeing this I remember telling them that things weren't imminent as I hadn't puked and that I always puked once I hit 7cm, so in my mind no puke meant no progress. They nodded with a knowing smile.

At around 4pm I felt something drop down out of me and was utterly convinced I'd had a serious uterine prolapse. I quickly realised this wasn't the case as I felt like someone was driving a flaming double decker bus through me at breakneck speed. I braced myself on the side of the pool and bit down hard (I left some rather impressive teeth marks in the liner!). One of the midwives told me that my baby's head had been born and that I should touch it. I told her I didn't want to touch it, thank you very much, and actually I didn't want to do this anymore so could they please push the head back up and stop it all. I considered asking to use the entonox at this point, and swore at myself for not going to hospital where I could have had an epidural.

Clearly a little concerned at the size of my baby the midwives told me to get on all fours, push hard and not scream – I didn't quite manage the not screaming part. I had to really work to push the baby's shoulders out – the head was out for quite a while before the next contraction – but when the rest of the body followed it came out in one huge contraction. At 4.13pm my baby landed on the pool floor looking very blue. I scooped him up and gave him a huge cuddle in shock that I had actually done it! I'd given birth with no intervention, no epidural, no pain relief and in a pool in my own home. Wow. I didn't need to look to see what we had when the midwife asked me if it was a girl or boy, as I had a hand full of squidgy warm testicles – Rafferty had arrived!

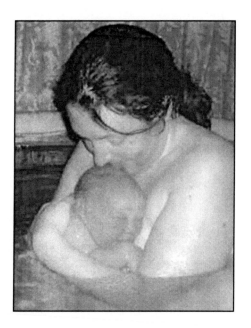

Around twenty minutes after the birth the pool started to get bloody and I really wanted to get out, so I was helped onto a duvet on the floor next to the pool. By this point the cord had long stopped pulsating so my husband (reluctantly) cut it, becoming only the second person to hold our little boy. We all took guesses at Rafferty's birth weight, and all agreed we thought he was in the mid 9lb range, so were very surprised when he tipped the scales at 11lb 3.5oz. Shortly after he was weighed one of the midwives showed me a text from the Head of Midwifery at the hospital congratulating us on our baby's birth and weight. I gather I was quite the topic of conversation for some time after.

Whilst the midwives cleaned everything up, I had a lovely hot lavender bath whilst my husband held Rafferty. By 6.30pm everybody had gone home and my other two children arrived back, eager to share their toys, over-enthusiastic hugs, kisses and drinks with the newest arrival. By 11pm we were all in bed, after the best-tasting curry I'd had in ages! I had finally had my much-needed, cathartic home water birth.

# Melissa Thomas

*Melissa Thomas planned to have her second baby unassisted. Her first daughter was born naturally in water at hospital. Her son arrived too quickly for the pool to be inflated, and here she describes how the bath can be equally as soothing and beneficial to birth. Melissa is a doula, breastfeeding peer supporter and advocate for human rights in childbirth.*

## Melissa's Story

My first experience of birth was truly empowering. After a reflective pregnancy I was afraid of labour, but during the process I managed to let go and embrace my instincts and I had a wonderful, natural water birth in hospital. It was the beginning of a healing journey that was a rite of passage. I learned a great deal about myself and my life in this time and I knew my second pregnancy would bring an end to this chapter and a new path to walk.

For my second pregnancy I opted to have minimum contact with maternity services and I began to consider freebirth. For me what appealed about the idea was the freedom and control it gave back to women and birth. I could imagine nothing more peaceful than allowing birth to take over with no interference. The more I thought about having midwives present, the more I felt it would be detrimental to my birthing experience.

I don't have a personal issue with midwives or hospitals. I think they do an amazing job under great pressure, but I don't believe that all women automatically need care in such a systematic way. It's great that we have these services for true emergencies, but more often than not this power can be abused and many women end up with a birth experience they find hard to process. I do not believe that birth belongs in a medical setting.

Birth should not be feared but embraced. I believe in a woman's ability to birth successfully provided she is surrounded by the right, supportive environment, one that she was able to make an informed decision about. Our bodies are designed to give life and this is a powerful, life-changing and emotional experience.

I do have strong opinions about birth, but I did not want my own experience to be caught up with this political aspect. I wasn't rejecting the system or trying to work against the grain, I just followed my instincts and trusted my choices. As my pregnancy progressed and I gained more knowledge I knew I would freebirth.

I did not have a specific due date as I had no ultrasound scans. I knew I was due sometime late September. On the morning of the 18th I woke up having mild contractions but by lunchtime they stopped. At 5pm I had a show and contractions started picking up again. They were very intense, coming every 20 minutes or so. They were just far enough apart to tease me into thinking I wasn't in labour, but just intense enough that I couldn't focus on anything else. At 8pm my partner David and I settled our daughter, Sofia, into bed. During this time the contractions became closer together but remained erratic.

I decided to run a bath. The idea of labouring in the bath appealed to me strongly: it had been very effective during my first birth. I was keen to know what it felt like to give birth outside of water, but this didn't seem right somehow. During my pregnancy I had even had a dream that I would give birth in the bath and I think somewhere inside I knew this wasn't far from the truth. I feel a pull towards water, I love the sea. When my husband and I first became partners he took me to a little fishing village on the North East coast and I found the ocean relaxing and restorative. The smell of the salty air, the crashing of waves, the ever-changing tide and the depth and breadth of the sea seem to have an incredible power that calms and heals. However, as my little bath tub filled up I began to feel extremely dizzy and sick. I could not get into the water and I didn't want to be alone. Labour appeared to be moving faster than I had anticipated. I was feeling afraid of the pain and so decided to contact our doula, Tina.

I followed my body's cues and feeling the need to be on all fours I knelt on the floor, resting against the bed, face down in the duvet. I used David's hand and leg to help me through contractions, pushing and squeezing while he held our daughter asleep on his other side. Time seemed to pass slowly and I didn't realise just how fast things were progressing. I was gradually feeling as though I was losing the ability to speak and all I could think about was water. I wanted to drink gallons of it and float motionless in it, feeling the warm, flowing sensation around me. I visualised myself alone in a stream, the water rippling. It was now approximately 11.30pm and David suggested I try the bath again. He topped it up with warm water. Sofia was awake by this point but she was relaxed too. As I tried to get up, I leaned back from all fours and the pain was intense. I rested against the wall unable to move. With David's help and a lot of concentration I eventually made it into the bath.

As soon as the water touched my skin I felt instant relief. As I lowered myself down the water transformed the sensations. I am almost unable to describe the feeling. It was a complete rush of oxytocin. I felt as though I was inside a bubble. My mind was completely clear and more in tune than ever before. I was aware of everything around me but I couldn't move and I couldn't speak. The contractions just came and went and I was completely still, silent and intently focused.It is one of the most powerful moments of my life.

When Tina arrived, David went to help her with the pool, leaving me alone in the bath. I thought about the idea of getting up, walking down the stairs and getting into the pool and it seemed like an impossible task. Then quite suddenly I heard a loud pop and a small gush of red came from between my legs followed by a stinging sensation. I lay back as I felt my body in complete control. A familiar sensation overtook me as I instinctively seemed to seize up and bear down. I let out a loud noise that I couldn't hold back. Tina came straight up to the bathroom and sat by my side holding my hand. We both knew my baby would be here soon. I still felt afraid and holding her hand helped me feel strong.

As I began to push my baby out I reached down to touch him. I felt the unmistakable feeling of his soft scalp and hair. With every push I could feel his whole body. It felt as though my body was moulding itself around his, easing him into the outside world. I felt excitement as his head appeared. I could feel our baby moving under water, half way between my body and the outside world. I began pushing again, his shoulders moved out and again a short pause before the rest of his body finally emerged in the water. I immediately lifted him up and put him to my chest. The rush of emotions and pure relief was incredible.

I remained in the bath for around an hour and a half, enjoying the refreshing feeling of the water, chatting with Tina and eating toast. I delivered the placenta in the toilet, then cut Oliver's cord. I rinsed and checked the placenta, keeping it to one side as I planned to encapsulate it myself.

Over time I will process this experience and place its meaning within the context of my life, as with my first birth. It feels like a true achievement – I have experienced something really special, a moment of absolute clarity, control and freedom in a world

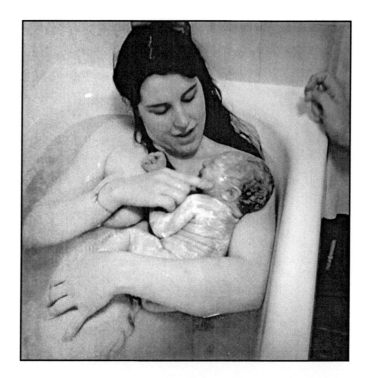

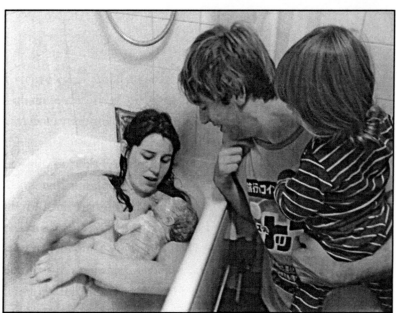

that frequently limits our choices and confines us within very narrow margins. It has been a journey that has opened my eyes to new perspectives about birth and life.

# Lucinda Story

*Lucinda Story lives with her daughter Willow in the market town of Stamford. Formerly a creative therapist and community artist, since motherhood Lucinda has been inspired to train as a babywearing consultant and Natal Hypnotherapy practitioner. Here she tells of how her exploration of her birth options ended in an outdoor water birth.*

## Lucinda's Story

*From fear to empowerment*

Through much of my pregnancy I allowed myself to dwell in a place of disempowerment. I was going through tough times: a strained relationship, challenging finances, and a move back to my family home. I initially dwelt in a place of intense fear, giving away the power I was born with as a woman designed to give birth. I looked to the medical profession and to glossy sensationalist magazines to educate me about pregnancy and birth, a topic I knew nothing about save for what I had learned in biology lessons at school.

A friend had mentioned using hypnosis for birth and when a second friend said she had a positive experience of this, I took it as a sign that it was right for me. I also came across some beautiful positive birth stories around this time, including a feature in the *Green Parent* magazine called 'Birthing in a Bender'. This inspired me to think outside the box in relation to where I wanted to birth. By this time my baby's father was also on board. We came across the Radical Midwives at a festival, and I went to learn what I could from their informal discussions. My eyes were opened to the idea of having a doula, and the benefits of having someone consistently present to support both partners. I also learnt much from the Radical Midwives about water birth.

## Queen of the waters

Willow was born head in water, body on land in October 2011 in a canvas bell tent situated in my parent's garden, close to two beautiful willow trees. This is my story of her birth.

I truly felt that all the midwives in attendance at my baby's birth (there was a change of midwives due to staffing issues) fully respected my birth preferences, which they had gone off to read by torchlight in a tent we had erected nearby. At one point during my labouring in the pool, I hit Willow's father with an inflatable pillow. On reflection I realise that this was 'transition'. This signified to the midwives that my baby was about to start birthing and they asked me to get out of the pool to have a wee. I tried to

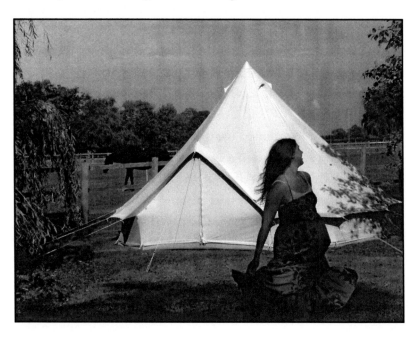

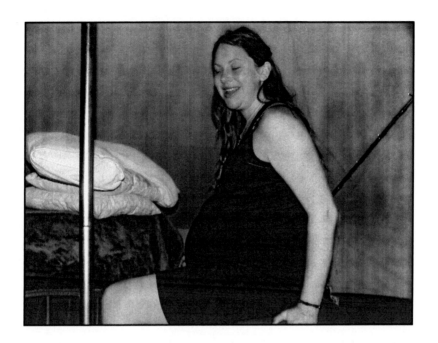

wee but nothing was coming out! I hadn't wanted to get out and I made a big fuss about it and accused the midwives of stressing me. I then agreed to a catheter* – a process I had always thought sounded really scary. The whole time, the midwives remained calm and confident, exuding a gentle quality. The catheter did not cause any discomfort – I was fine, and able to get back into the pool and commence the final part of Willow's journey now that a full bladder no longer blocked her path.

In getting out of the water, I had come up a little out of a deep hypnotic state and was more externally focused than before. In a lucid state, I remember a running commentary I gave the midwives who were respectfully keeping a little distance, kneeling on our makeshift bed, trusting me to birth intuitively. 'What should I do?', I asked. 'I could bear down but I don't feel an overwhelming urge to'. I verbalised the details of this stage of my labour; where my baby's head was in the birth canal, how it came down and then back up a little. The analytical thinking part of my brain, the neo-cortex, grasped onto the idea of the ring of fire. I awaited this moment and thankfully it never came. I felt a strong sensation but in no way could it be described as a ring of fire! I felt no pain from the birthing part of my labour, only joy and calm. As I closed my eyes, focusing inward, an image of the two willow trees only metres away came into my mind. My body was showing signs of tiredness after 36 hours of labour. My feet kept slipping from under me as I pulled myself up to squat, holding on to the handles in my birth pool. I was grateful for the support the water gave in helping me to hold my heavy body up.

My baby and I were on the cusp of a huge transition for us both, from womb to world, from maiden to mother. The endorphins and oxytocin released with a massive love for my baby, and the excitement of being on the cusp of greeting her, transcended the sensations of my body's contractions. My baby's head was crowning; one of the midwives said I could touch it, but I questioned her as I had thought it might encourage my baby to take her first breath too soon. After being reassured that it was 'safe' to do so, I recall the magical moment of connection between two worlds as my fingers met the jelly-like consistency of my baby's fontanelle. I then very gently helped my skin to stretch around her head. Time stood still.

My baby's head had been born. From the watery world inside me, I could feel my baby flipping like a dolphin in her attempts to swim down into the larger water world around her head. This sensation amazed and excited me. The two midwives, now kneeling by the pool, calmly told me when I had my next contraction, 'Lucinda, we'd like you to step out of the pool please.' After saying I couldn't and asking a few nonsensical questions, I stepped easily out of the pool aided by the hand of a midwife, head dangling between legs. I knelt on all fours. The cord had been around my baby's neck, holding her in a half-birthed state – this was slipped aside (unbeknown to me) by one of the midwives and my baby flopped out just like that. Greeted by her father with 'Hello Willow'.

Time continued to stand still whilst we waited for Willow's first breath. I paused, engulfed by calm and a sense of trust in the midwives – strangers who had trusted me – as they suctioned Willow's lungs. I knew my baby was here now and that she would be OK. A few moments later and Willow was in my arms, wrapped in a blanket I had arranged for our doula to pre-warm on the electric radiator heating the bell tent. I looked into her eyes, glassy and directionless as we met, sixteen days after her estimated delivery date. She marked me as her territory by pooing on me. I had anticipated that I would cry at this point – I didn't, rather I felt a deep and content peace. Willow

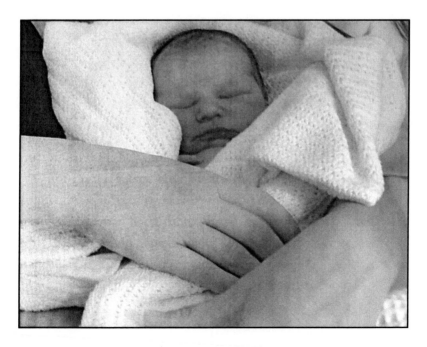

was passed to her father, whom she punched (apparently known as breast-boxing) whilst I was supported in squatting to birth the placenta that had previously acted as Willow's life support. The cord had been cut as it ceased to pulsate, which I had outlined in my birth preferences.

## Comfort measures

My two main pain relief methods were birth hypnosis and water. I used various other comfort measures such as massage, a birth ball, dance and homeopathy. At no point was I at all tempted to ask for medical pain relief. The use of water was definitely appropriate for me. I made the classic mistake of getting in the pool too early and not wanting to have to get out and feel the weight of my heavy labouring body again. It's possible that this may have slowed labour down a little, but equally there were other factors that could have come into play.

Once things had reached a climax of intensity and we all knew that Willow was on her way out, the pool was amazing! I rocked from side to side, creating waves to massage around my middle through contractions. The warmth and weaker gravitational pull from within the pool comforted me immensely. The physical boundaries of the pool combined with hypnosis provided me with a protective bubble in which to enter my birthing body. I have no regrets about anything related to Willow's birth.

# Sarah Berryman

*Sarah Berryman's first baby was born at home in the birthing pool. After hoping for the same for her second child, her pregnancy took an unexpected turn and she ended up having an emergency caesarean. Here she tells of how 'rebirthing' in water helped her emotional healing following her son's difficult birth. Sarah lives near Derby with her husband, three-year-old daughter, and baby son.*

## A Tale of Two Births... and one Rebirth

March 2013: the month my world turned upside-down. The country was covered in a rare spring snow, and my son, for whom we had planned a calm home water birth, was born.

My waterbirthing story begins more than three years earlier, when I was pregnant with our daughter Lydia. I don't remember when, or why, I chose to plan a home water birth – it was just something that had 'been there' as long as I remember. It was never a choice between hospital or home; home was my natural choice and I never wavered from that. Overall, Lydia's pregnancy was smooth and positive – I made an informed decision to decline dates-based induction and my contractions started when I was just past 42 weeks pregnant.

After over 50 hours of strong but manageable contractions, I climbed into the birthing pool. The water helped me stay calm, took the edge off my contractions, which were almost on top of each other by this point, and, best of all, being in my little blue inflatable pool made me feel as if I was in my own private 'birthing bubble', which gave me privacy despite the two midwives nearby. I leant on the side of the pool, holding my husband Ben's hands throughout. After less than an hour and a half in the pool, my little waterbaby Lydia was in my arms, born at 42 weeks and three days and weighing exactly seven and a half pounds. I got out of the pool to deliver her placenta – I had planned to deliver the placenta naturally, but ended up having a managed third stage due to concerns over blood loss. Half an hour after Lydia's birth I was sitting on the sofa, with my husband, and Lydia was breastfeeding for the very first time.

Two and a half years later, after overcoming fertility issues and recurrent miscarriages, we were overjoyed to find out we were pregnant with our longed for second child. Having had an easy pregnancy and birth previously, I naturally hoped for, and to some extent probably expected, the same second time round. I was healthy, well informed, had an incredibly positive approach to birth, and we also had an Independent Midwife* to support us. What could possibly go wrong?

\* \* \* \* \*

Unfortunately the reality was rather different. Our little 'Starbaby' had a rocky pregnancy; heavy bleeding from a haemorrhage in my womb in the first trimester, and in the second, talipes (club foot), a two-vessel cord and possible growth restriction and low fluid diagnosed via ultrasound. We were seen regularly in the Fetal Medicine Unit, and our wonderful Independent Midwife Jo came with us to every appointment. During the third trimester things seemed to be looking more positive; Starbaby was growing steadily (although he was still small), my fluid levels were apparently up, and his heart, kidneys etc all seemed perfect at every ultrasound. We decided to plan for another home water birth, with a low hospital transfer threshold should there be any concerns at any point.

At 36 weeks we had our 'wet run' with the birthing pool, which brought happy memories of Lydia's birth flooding back. She repeatedly asked, 'Please may you pretend to give birth to me, Mummy?' and I was happy to oblige. The feeling of the bottom of the inflatable pool on my knees, the sight of the floating thermometer... everything triggered wonderful memories of three years earlier. I desperately hoped that our little boy would be born in the same pool as his sister, with just his parents, sister and Jo there.

However, our life as a family was about to take a different path. I was just past 39 weeks pregnant when I felt Starbaby's movements slow. He had a normal pattern of a few active days followed by a few quiet days... but this 'quiet day' felt different. My instincts told me that something wasn't right. I listened to his heartbeat with the Doppler we had bought to reassure ourselves after our very first miscarriage, and it was beating fast, much faster than normal. I heard his heart rate suddenly drop right down before gradually climbing up again and knew I needed to call Jo. She came straight over to our house and listened to his heartbeat, and we heard two more decelerations. That 'low transfer threshold' that we hoped we'd never need, was coming into play. Jo and I drove to hospital while Ben stayed at home for now, as Lydia was fast asleep in bed. A CTG showed our little boy was in major (and increasing) distress, and I made the only choice I could, to have an emergency caesarean. Ben made it to hospital just in time, and our precious boy Jasper was born soon after. He weighed a little over five and a half pounds, was very floppy and covered with thick meconium, inside and out. It scares me to think about it, but I know we got him out just in time.

An emergency caesarean was clearly the polar opposite of everything we hoped for in Jasper's birth. Instead of coming into the world in a warm birthing pool at home, he was plucked from me in a bright, unfamiliar operating theatre. Despite knowing I was making the right decision, it was the scariest night of my life – our little boy was so, so close to not surviving. Jasper spent eight days in NICU before we were finally able to come home where we belong.

My midwife Jo suggested that we might like to consider having a 'rebirth' for Jasper in the birthing pool once we had settled back at home. My initial reaction was skeptical – why would I want to remind myself of the gentle birth that Jasper and I could no longer have? I worried that it would be too upsetting to be in the birthing pool, knowing I could never give birth to him in there. For a while after his birth, I felt like I was still waiting to give birth to him, and I wasn't sure whether getting back in the pool would help or hinder my emotional recovery from such a traumatic time.

I decided, though, to go into it with an open mind. Nine days after we came home from hospital, Ben and Lydia inflated and filled the pool just as they had planned to do when I went into labour. I climbed into the pool and instantly felt calm and happy. Jo undressed Jasper, Ben passed him to me in the pool... and seconds after touching the water, Jasper fell fast asleep. Lydia joined us in the water and we spent some time cuddling, talking about her birth, and sharing what our hopes had been for Jasper's birth. We listened to (and I cried to) the special songs I had hoped to give birth to and I whispered some words to Jasper that I had written that morning. I told him we had hoped he would be born in this birthing pool, but that he had shown me he needed something different and I had listened to him. I said that we wanted him to know the feeling of being held in gentle, loving arms in a warm birthing pool, surrounded by love. I repeated a line that Ben and I had written into our wedding vows nearly

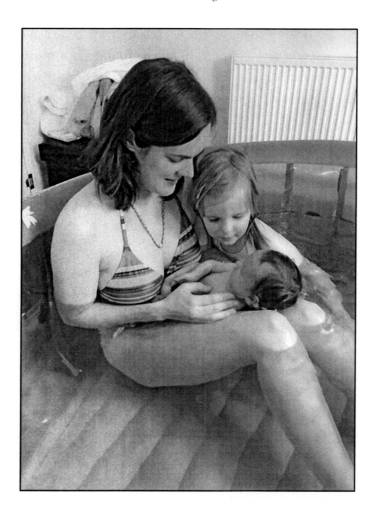

seven years earlier – 'We will catch you if you fall and help you live your dreams'.

As the water started to cool, we climbed out and dried ourselves off, then all snuggled together on the sofa. I breastfed Jasper in the exact spot where Lydia had had her first breastfeed and we all feasted on Jasper's '0th birthday cake', which Ben and Lydia had baked and decorated (with stars) that morning. A wonderful end to a beautiful experience for us all.

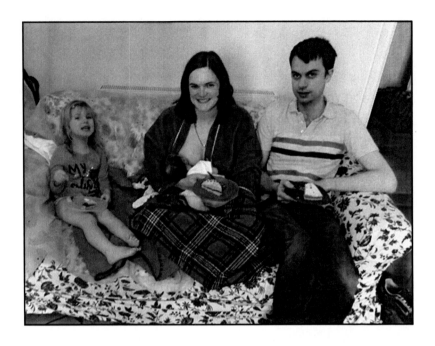

My initial worries about 'rebirthing' Jasper had left me, and although it was an emotional and at times sad experience, I know I will forever be glad that we got the birthing pool back out and spent that precious time giving Jasper a calm, wonderful rebirth. From that day on, I have felt like I have two water-babies. Jasper's birth and the surrounding events were incredibly difficult, and will always be a part of me. But alongside those memories I will now forever be able to think back to how he slept in my arms in the birthing pool for over an hour, how he seemed more relaxed in the water than at any other time in the sixteen days he had been in this world, and how I looked down at my precious, miracle boy and started to believe for the first time that the emotional wounds from his birth and early days might one day heal.

# Chloe Smee

*Chloe Smee had her second baby at home after an untidy hospital transfer during her first labour. Thanks to a fantastic doula and birth partner, lots of preparation and a robust birth pool, the birth was a healing and humane experience, which Chloe wishes every woman could have. Chloe lives with her husband and two children in York and is the chair of a local food charity.*

## Frieda is born

Sitting here writing with a seventeen-week old Frieda slumbering on her sheepskin bed next to me, it is ridiculous to imagine a world before her, a world without her, a world in which she wasn't at the beginning and end of every thought. Even more, to remember the anxiety that we carried before her birth. Her brother Noah's birth had been a violent eruption that cleaved me open, puncturing a peaceful pregnancy and leaving me unsure of foot as I took my first steps into motherhood. Frieda's birth, by contrast, created a fluid passage between the pregnancy and the life that followed.

The pregnancy stretched into the 41st week, and the calmness of mind I had been nurturing was being tested. The house grew busy as we loaded the freezer and cleaned frenetically for our new baby. The arrival of Supergran afforded me more rest, but created an atmosphere of heightened expectation which threatened to destroy my carefully-nurtured zen-mind. Waiting for a baby's arrival is utterly unique. Not just the lack of control, but the feeling of being so near to something so completely mysterious, yet so intimately known. And which will revolutionise your life in total, yet unknown ways.

The night before the labour, I broke emotionally: I can see now that this release was the start of the labour process. And that evening I augmented things further: sitting by a fire in the garden with my love and a glass of red wine; putting headphones on and grinding low to some deep reggae; making love in the wee small hours (it's hard to remember now, but that last phase of pregnancy was sex, sex, sex – a far cry from life with a baby).

Later I woke with a vague sense of movement in my womb. At around 3am I was confident enough to give the sensations their name, and voice the happy news that labour was beginning. This quiet, unhurried start and the sheer joy I felt helped me to create a protected bubble for the birth that was – pretty much – impenetrable. It was dark. I felt quiet. There was no urgency. Just the need to prompt Nik, with every contraction, to press deep into my lower back (both my babies were back-to-back), while I immersed myself in the deep, deep breathwork I had been rehearsing for months (after a weirdly disembodied experience during Noah's birth, I had prioritised deep yoga and meditation practices during my second pregnancy: I was in serious training!).

And we dozed on and off. At 5ish, Nik roused himself to set up the birth pool, and arrange the plethora of towels and plastic sheets. He also had an Irish coffee to steady his nerves! I continued in the dark, quiet world of the bedroom, pressing my lower back into a stack of hardback books I'd positioned against the wall in lieu of Nik's warm hands. At some point, I needed to be in a more alert, upright mode. My body called me to squat deep and low against a cool leather chair with every contraction, and spontaneous low grunts accompanied my breathing. The breath kept me calm, free from any questioning or panicking, and created a point of focus and strength through each short contraction. To fully let each contraction go, I adopted the technique of releasing a very long, deep breath at the close of each contraction and whispering, 'thank you'. With this simple practice (inspired by Gurmurkh*), I was able to retain a sense of wonder at the everyday miracle my body was participating in and to remember the baby – my baby – travelling down to my arms. All of this sounds a bit high-minded when written down – but it was so acutely real during the labour. Such simple, repeated statements as, 'let go', 'thank you' and 'move into the pain' truly kept my mind in my body and on the job. (The idea of 'moving into the pain' was the most useful reminder: the experience of the contractions had me instinctually rearing away from the pain, in a vain attempt to escape it. Instead, moving into the pain meant seeing where the contraction wanted my body to go – using the contraction as a message to help the labour).

A while later, Nik reappeared, strengthened by his Irish breakfast, suggesting we rouse Mum so that she could carry Noah into the day's adventures. A joyful sense of busy preparation spread throughout the house, while I stayed in the womb of our bedroom and in the womb of my breath, attending to each contraction. Noah, however, had other ideas. Elated at the news the baby was on its way, he wanted to come and join me – and I wanted him too. He bustled in, all night-time hair-scruff, crumpled and hot. There was no time to think about how I would work my contractions in his company. But my contractions, miraculously, calmed right down, allowing me to fully give myself to cuddling my beautiful boy and hearing the story he'd brought in to me.

As the family moved off into the day, I stayed upstairs, moving between the bedroom and the bathroom. And when I moved, how the contractions strengthened! The contractions I experienced when moving to the loo had me gripping the side of the bath on my knees, knocked by the intensity. But still the breath work kept me calm. I kept telling myself 'I can do it' – in contrast to the messages the midwives had given me during Noah's birth. During this time I stepped into the shower a couple of times, which brought things on harder and faster, but equally things were soothed immeasurably by the flowing water.

During my third shower – I needed to feel water but wanted to delay my entrance to the pool and stay as active as possible – I felt the labour intensify considerably. I was so immersed in the physical experience of the labour that I spontaneously reached down and gave myself what amounted to a vaginal examination (VE). We had decided to have no VEs throughout the labour – they seemed so intrusive, and to encourage an unnecessary obsession with a model of labour 'progress' which is informed by graphs, not the labouring mother or baby. This experience, of feeling my cervix open and even the warmth of my new baby's head wrapped in its amniotic sac, was other-worldly. The tangibility made everything so much more acute. Whether caused by the profundity of feeling my baby's head or the physical push this gave to my cervix, my labour leapt forward. Nik called Hannah, Superdoula, who had been making preparations to come over, and I made my way to the birth pool, feeling the need for some more pain-relief and support.

The next phase of the labour took place in the intimate environment of the birth pool, where I was immersed from about 1pm. Although it was a bright sunshiny day, the pool felt calm and dark and was a further guard against me engaging with the things that were going on around me – the passing of time, the needs of Nik and Hannah, the unexpected intrusion of a midwife into the proceedings. I tried to keep well away from the clocks. Any time I veered towards, 'How long will this last?', or

'How long was that contraction?', or 'How long has this been going on for?', Nik and Hannah brought me back to my body.

With their support, my self-belief snowballed. And it needed to, because the contractions were getting harder and I was getting wobbly and tired. I started getting hot and cold, and my self-doubt started emerging. I stayed with the mantras – I knew that I had to fight the fear that was rising in me. I can now see these are all classic signs of 'transition', but I couldn't see it at the time. I needed a change of scene, and got out of the pool. I was really struggling now. The contractions were hard and fast and images of being stuck in this phase for hours kept invading my mind.

Outside of the pool, there was no escape from this intensity. Between contractions, I apologised to Nik and Hannah, saying we needed to abandon plan A and get to the hospital for an epidural – I couldn't carry on like this. They kindly ignored my pleas. Hannah calmly passed me a cloth infused with essential oils, which I managed to breathe in, although I was enraged at this pathetic excuse for a spinal anaesthetic.

Amidst the anger and the disbelief and the fear that were rising in me, my baby was about ready to emerge. The intensity is indescribable. Heat, chaos, panic, fear, acute pain, studied breathwork – and all somehow continuing in an atmosphere of care and calm. My mind suddenly disengaged, as if to help me get to the next level, my hips spontaneously engaged in a ferocious wiggle (accompanied by Cesaria Evora on the stereo), and I started roaring, 'Yes! Yes! Yes!'

And as I shouted, my mind completely cleared, as if a storm had passed. I felt complete clarity, and freedom from pain, and I knew with absolute certainty that it was time to push. Hannah dashed outside to call Team Midwife and I dashed to the pool (at least, it felt like a dash) with Nik's help.

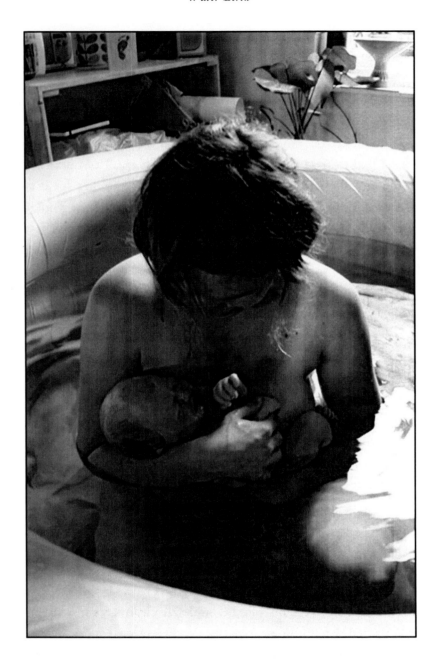

The final phase is a blur. I remember deep, guttural noises emerging from me. I remember being thrilled that I was ready to push. I remember the freedom of movement in the water. I remember a flurry of midwives arriving and the careful calm we'd nurtured being punctured – but I was beyond caring. I was nearing the end. I was elated. I loved the feeling of being able to push – I knew exactly what to do. I loved the feeling of power and pushed harder than was probably wise. I was doing it! With one final roar I felt the ultimate stretch... and suddenly there was a head between my legs. This feels at least as surreal as it sounds: suddenly everything seemed to stop. In this final phase, you can only push with the power of a contraction behind you. I knelt there, in the pool, with a baby's head between my legs for what felt like hours. And I knew the hard work was over, even though I didn't have a baby in my arms quite yet.

Then a sudden wave carried the final contraction through my body and with a calm slither I felt our blessed wee baby emerge. Nik caught this fresh, slippery creature and brought it up through my legs and into my waiting arms. So with tears of total gratitude I held baby Frieda's being, eyes tight shut, arms flailing in their new-found freedom, in my gaze. And that's where she stays, still now, at the centre of my gaze, held in total gratitude. My little girl.

Of course the story doesn't end there. There was a first feed in the pool, with its lazy latch. There was the placenta rushing out as I made my exit (expertly caught in a washing-up bowl by Nik). There were stitches on the sofa, which I received gleefully, in the afterglow of our birth. There were midwives complaining about the lack of data for their forms (as they'd arrived so late on in the process). There was Noah, returning home with Granny to complete our little family. There was the four of us in bed together in a sleepless haze, Frieda complaining about the lack of proper milk, Noah complaining about her noise. There we are – the four of us. Complete. Completed, by the arrival in the world of our little girl, Frieda Betty.

# Françoise Freedman

*In parallel with her academic career as a medical anthropologist at Cambridge University, Françoise Freedman is the founder of Birthlight. She has developed body-based innovative methods of prenatal education, birth attendance and parent-baby interaction, drawn in part on her background as a swimmer and yoga therapist and in part on her field research in the Peruvian Upper Amazon. A pioneer of Aquanatal Yoga, Françoise has particularly enjoyed exploring the power of water to facilitate the birth process in its physical, physiological and spiritual aspects.*

## Françoise's stories

Many water births flash through my memory as I sit down to write. Intense emotions come with each birth scene, with a replay of sensations that are singularly more vivid than those of dry births. Does water affect not just the birth process as women experience it, but also the whole scene of birth? We still know so little about the emotional conductivity of water, even with Masaro Emotu's remarkable work. For many years I have helped pregnant women to practise push-glides in shallow pools or dive-glides in deeper pools, finding the release of movement in their bodies as they relax more and more, letting out air slowly in extended exhalations. Invariably, women report that the memory of this practice carried through to their labour, facilitating their transition to the second stage.

Water helps birthing women to find their spontaneous breathing rhythm, as their bodies require, just as in a full yoga breath, particularly when immersed to shoulder level. Breathing takes on an ebb and flow of waves, each different from the next. Voiced breaths and sounds take on a different quality, as if the water took them in without muffling them. In turn, the sounds of water as women move, or when sprinkled or poured or trickled, seem to affect everyone present. Michel Odent often remarks on the calming effect of traditional kettle-boiling activities on attendants and birth partners at home births, and on the power of simply turning a tap on to activate labour.

Two births I attended still fill me with wonder to this day about the sensory quality of emotions that water helps release during birth. In the first, I acted as birth attendant for a woman in hospital at her request because her Chinese husband did not consider it appropriate for him to be with her. I was aware of his presence in the waiting room, with a huge bunch of two dozen red roses. After a few hours, contractions were steady but progress was slow. I was familiar with this 6cm hitch, often associated with mental or psychological hurdles, and suggested we make our way to one of the small bathrooms as there was still no water birth facility in Cambridge at the time.

The memory of this bathroom is so vivid that I shift to the present tense. Anxious to fill the bath as quickly as possible while Nora leans forward against the wall, I turn both taps to the full. This triggers not only a set of powerful contractions, but also a cascade of loud sobbing, shriek crying to screaming pitch, followed by uncontrollable bouts of laughter that I cannot help joining in unwittingly. Loud bangs at the door follow. 'What's going on in there, get out!' I reply that all is fine, and let the midwife in to check. The sounds coming out of the bathroom have clearly caused uproar. It's a busy night on the labour ward. Nora's labour seems to pause as she settles in the bath. Now we are alone again and her emotional roller coaster takes off with a vengeance as I pour water on her back. Bits of opera, roaring laughter again, a vocal gamut ranging from the depths of despair to clouds of bliss leaves me in awe of the female psyche. Looking back, it was probably the wildest orgasmic birth I have ever witnessed, but this was not in my awareness at the time. The memory of the moment when I realized that the baby's head was crowning and I stood at the cusp between acting responsibly and pulling the emergency cord, or just letting it happen, is forever with me.

I did pull the cord, opened the door, saw the wheelchair approaching, and lifted a now surprisingly silent Nora into the wheelchair with the help of a new midwife to zoom her to one of the rooms across the passage. The baby girl was born on the towels as we both lifted Nora from the wheelchair, in an improvised supported squat before we could hoist her onto the bed. A senior midwife and a junior registrar witnessed the scene and soon we were all laughing and crying with Nora. Neither the junior registrar nor the younger midwife, who was from the Caribbean, had seen a totally spontaneous delivery before. They hugged as if to comfort each other. The midwife said that this moment was her dream, her reason for becoming a midwife. After an uneventful sequence of re-owning the hospital post-birth process, as though the bathroom episode had never happened, Nora's husband was called in and brought his roses.

The second scene that emerges in my mind to conjure up how water mediates emotions in a peculiar way in water birth is very different. It's one of many romantic and zany idyllic water births I attended in the late 1980s and early 1990s. Couples from all walks of life, yet all somewhat eccentric, sought brave midwives to care for them in their homes at a time when birthing pools were not yet available. We made do with a home water tank that a resourceful dad equipped with in-flowing and out-flowing hoses, one blue and one red, with great copper valves. I delivered the tank on the roof rack of my car, with my children holding it down through the windows.

Looking at this rather horrible black tank that is now the watering source for our greenhouse, still with the names of babies engraved on it, I marvel at how pioneer water birthers put up with such discomfort. They did so because water made them feel that they could let go and be free. Images of ocean births started to spread around and it was still in the early days of underwater photography. Within the confines of the tank – which a consultant referred to as my 'bucket', along with an invitation to take out the best insurance money could buy – women found privacy, freedom and release. Candlelight was a must-have and there was an awareness of the season, of the animals that were drawn to the event, of the rhythms of the day and night.

In this instance as in others, Harriet laboured silently by herself while her husband Ralf, the two midwives and I stood back. Now and again she looked up for Ralf, who sat a little way from the tank, and their loving non-verbal exchange took Harriet through the next bit of labour. She invited my teenage daughter, who had come with me to be with her two small children in case they woke up, to witness her birth. Between the flickering candle and the first glimmers of dawn, the flux of the water around her moving body and the gentle rain on the roof and trees around, the crackling wood fire in the hearth and our team support around the tub, Harriet was in her zone. She was in charge of what was clearly not an easy labour with a personal courage that reminded me of the way I had seen rainforest women give birth to their babies in the Amazon region. Just as in the rainforest, the very experienced midwife monitored the process with minimal interference and few words.

My daughter and I were bonded anew in the rich silence of this shared experience. When the little one appeared, it was a moment of initiation that I wish many other teenage girls could experience. There was no space for fear, not because Harriet and her experienced midwife were not aware that complications might arise, but because the water in the tank-tub provided a containing, protecting space in which birth could be anticipated as safe and a part of life rather than deemed normal in retrospect.

*It is said that women in labour leave their bodies. They travel to the stars to collect the souls of their babies, and return to this world together.*

**Anon**

# Epilogue

During the long, slow, stop-start labour of editing this book, I have had another water baby. I'm not going to tell you his birth story – perhaps you have heard enough – but I am going to tell you about a healing experience that I did not anticipate, in this, my second experience of giving birth in water.

When I had my first baby in a hospital induction, I think this created some difficult feelings between myself and the man I love. I was traumatised by the experience, and no doubt he was too. Perhaps he felt he had let me down, and perhaps I felt let down by him, or even that I had let him down by not birthing easily and naturally as I had told him I would.

They must be quite common, these dark treacly feelings that lurk and stick in those days, weeks and months after a difficult birth.

Much focus is on the baby, and there is little time to discuss what happened. Although we did try, I suspect that some of those difficult feelings lingered in the shadows and came out in a variety of mischievous and downright unpleasant ways.

My second birth (and first water birth) was in many ways a very selfish experience. I really needed to prove to myself that I could conquer my many fears and birth my baby unaided. In the protecting circle of the birth pool, I did just that, and once my baby was in my arms, I remember repeating, 'I did it! I did it!'.

My partner was of course present for that birth, and I felt deeply and madly in love with him that day, but my main support during the labour came from the female midwife who attended me.

It was as if some trust had been lost in that first birth and I needed to 'go it alone' this time. This birth was extremely healing and empowering – for me – but perhaps not for 'us'.

My third and final birth was different. At the suggestion of our midwife, my man and I spent a few hours alone in the birth pool as I laboured, lit by candles and listening to beautiful Joni Mitchell sing.

Allowing my man into the water with me felt rather like a Queen allowing someone into her innermost circle. Often in modern birth the woman is the permission-seeker, but water birth upends this. The woman reigns, and if anyone wants to do anything to her or with her, they have to ask nicely, or get wet, or both.

In the darkness and stillness of night we floated there together, and the waters brought healing of a different kind: a cleansing of past traumas and regrets, and a reunification of the masculine and feminine that culminated in a baby boy popping up to the surface of the water like a celebratory cork from a bottle.

Of course, as I write this we are now deep into the blurry sleep-deprived phase of our son's babyhood, barely connecting with each other as we struggle to survive the crazy first year of life with a small and utterly dependent human – that as well as the other two wombats with their energy, their tantrums, their spillages, their beautiful chaos.

But I like to think that when we meet again on the other side, something of that time in the water will resurface, a deep memory of that moment of healing, a recollection of a reconnection.

We cannot predict what birth will bring, nor what water birth will bring. Both are full of surprises and that is both their beauty and their power. What we can say for certain is that by choosing water birth we are inviting birth to be empowering, healing, and transformative.

And birth is very likely to answer our invitation, as we float, struggle and triumph in our ultimate sanctuary, our watery nest, our big dark skirts... our circle full of water.

# Glossary

**AIMS**

Association for Improvements in Maternity Services, see Resources.

**Allow/allowed**

Sometimes women feel that decisions in pregnancy and labour are taken out of their hands; however, it is important to remember that you are able to exercise your own judgement to make informed choices; you have a human right to have your baby how and where you choose; decisions are yours to make. For more see:

- *www.birthrights.org.uk*
- *www.humanrightsinchildbirth.com*

**Amni-hook**

Instrument similar to a crochet hook used to break the bag of amniotic fluid surrounding the baby, sometimes to induce or speed up labour.

**Birth pool**

Several different types available for home/hospital use - see 'Resources'.

**Braxton Hicks**

'Practice' contractions felt prior to labour – may be quite strong! Can be felt from around 20 to 30 weeks onwards; distinguished from labour by the fact that they don't increase in intensity or frequency. Some mothers don't experience them at all, others have them a lot. If in doubt, ask your midwife!

**Catheter**

A flexible tube inserted into the bladder to drain urine.

**Colostrum**

First milk produced by a mother's breasts; may leak out before the birth. Highly concentrated and packed with antibodies, it is often referred to as 'liquid gold', partly due to its colour (yellowish) and partly due to its importance for the baby's gut health. All the food a healthy newborn needs in the first few days.

## Episiotomy

A cut made in the perineum by a midwife or doctor to increase the size of the vaginal opening and allow the baby to be born quickly. Not performed routinely; usually needed for instrumental (forceps/ventouse) delivery.

## Foetus ejection reflex

Spontaneous rapid birth without conscious or directed pushing on the part of the mother. Described by Michel Odent as occurring naturally if the conditions at birth are right (dark, safe, trusted companions).

## Gurmurkh

Gurmukh Kaur Khalsa is a teacher of Kundalini Yoga and a pioneer in the field of prenatal yoga. She has published several books and DVDs.

## GTT

Glucose Tolerance Test. Used to diagnose gestational diabetes in the mother, which may mean she is more likely to have a large baby. Some mothers decline the test based on their personal circumstances; if you are concerned about it, do your own research.

## Ina May

Ina May Gaskin, American midwife and birth activist, author of influential birth books *Spiritual Midwifery* and *Ina May's Guide to Childbirth*.

## Independent Midwife/IM

Self-employed midwife who provides care outside the NHS, paid for privately by parents. They can offer one-to-one care throughout pregnancy and birth, and support parents to access their choices even in difficult circumstances (e.g. twin home birth, breech birth). See 'Resources'.

## Induction/induce

Starting labour early, usually for a pregnancy that has gone 'post-dates'. Medical methods include prostaglandin gels and pessaries, syntocin drips and artificial rupture of membranes (ARM), and membrane 'sweeps'. More 'natural' methods, e.g. acupuncture, castor oil etc still encourage labour to start before the body may be ready. Induced labours can be more intense or painful. Some feel that induction for post-dates is unnecessary and that babies will come when they are ready; others have concerns about longer pregnancies. Careful research can help you make an informed decision.

## Macrosomia
The medical term for a big baby, weighing more than 4.5kg / 9lb 15oz at birth.

## Meconium
A baby's first bowel movement, sometimes a sign that the baby has been or is becoming distressed. Can be harmful to the baby if it is breathed in; caregivers thus tend to be cautious if it is observed.

## Moxibustion
A traditional Chinese medicine therapy used to encourage breech babies to turn head down, which involves the burning of herbs near to the body.

## PGP
Pelvic Girdle Pain, formerly known as SPD (Symphysis Pubis Disorder): severe pain from adjustments in the alignment of the bones of the pelvis during pregnancy. May make it hard to be mobile or find comfortable positions in labour.

## Plug
Mucous in the cervix that comes away when the cervix begins to dilate, often signalling that labour will begin soon. Has the appearance of heavy vaginal discharge or a jelly-like substance, may be blood-stained.

## Pre-eclampsia
Complication of pregnancy characterised by high blood pressure, and protein in the urine. Risk of serious complications to mother and baby means that careful monitoring followed by birth by induction or caesarean is usually necessary.

## Third stage
The phase of birth in which the placenta is delivered, after the baby is born.

## VE
Optional vaginal examination, performed to check the dilation of the cervix.

# Resources

## Organisations

### Birthrights
Organisation promoting and defending UK women's human rights in childbirth
*www.birthrights.org*

### Tell Me a Good Birth Story
This group will match you with a 'birth buddy' to inspire you with information and positivity
*www.tellmeagoodbirthstory.com*

### The Positive Birth Movement
Global network of free antenatal discussion groups
*www.positivebirthmovement.org*

### Active Birth
A yoga-based approach to labour and birth
*www.activebirthcentre.com*

### Association for Improvements in the Maternity Services (AIMS)
Information and support for all birth choices
*www.aims.org.uk*

### Doula UK
Professional birth companions to offer information, support and advocacy
*www.doula.org.uk*

### Which? Birth Choice
Information to help you choose where to have your baby
*www.which.co.uk/birth-choice*

## Association of Radical Midwives

Supporting those who wish to give or receive personalised maternity care

*www.midwifery.org.uk*

## Campaign for Normal Birth

RCM Campaign to inspire and support normal birth practice

*www.rcmnormalbirth.org.uk*

## Home Birthers and Hopefuls

Support and information for those planning to birth at home, with an active Facebook page

*www.homebirthersandhopefuls.com*

## Home Birth Reference Site

Goldmine of info on home birth, with an active Yahoo discussion group

*www.homebirth.org.uk*

## Independent Midwives

Qualified and regulated midwives working outside of the NHS

*www.independentmidwives.org.uk*

## Birthlight

Charity and teacher-training organisation focusing on the holistic approach to pregnancy, birth and babyhood

*www.birthlight.co.uk*

## Natal Hypnotherapy

Information about using hypnotherapy for pregnancy and birth

*www.natalhypnotherapy.co.uk*

## BIRTH POOL HIRE

There are a wealth of pools for sale or hire if you search online. Most popular is the inflatable variety such as:

*www.birthpoolinabox.co.uk*

You might wish to consider hiring a heated and filtered pool. This means you can have it filled and ready to go well in advance of labour.

*www.bornathome.co.uk*

# BOOKS ABOUT WATER BIRTH

**Out of print but worth tracking down in online bookstores:**

*The Water Birth Book*, Janet Balaskas

*Water and Sexuality*, Michel Odent, Arkana 1990

*Choosing Waterbirth: Reclaiming the Sacred Power of Birth*, Lakshmi Bertram

*Water Birth Unplugged: Proceedings of the First International Water Birth Conference*, ed. Beverley A. Lawrence Beech, Books for Midwives Press 1996

**In print:**

*Revisiting Water Birth, an attitude to care*, Dianne Garland, Palgrave Macmillan 2010

*Water Birth: A Midwives Perspective*, Susanna Napierala, Praeger 1994

*The Heart in the Womb*, Amali Lokugamage, Docamali 2011

(For children) *Our Water Baby*, A. MacLean & J. Nesbitt, The Good Birth Company 2007

# Also available from Lonely Scribe

## HOME BIRTHS
### stories to inspire and inform

A moving collection of real life stories celebrating the joy and wonder of birth at home. This collection of first-hand recollections by mothers and their partners gives an insight into the modern experience of home birth, from the first decision to the final push.

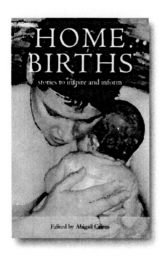

**ISBN 978-1-905179-02-2**

**£13.99/$24.99**

## BREASTFEEDING
### stories to inspire and inform

This collection of first-hand accounts by mothers aims to educate and inspire anyone wondering how to feed their new baby. The real-life stories of other women are hugely empowering for those who may be struggling with getting breastfeeding established or keeping going.

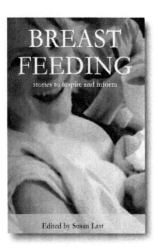

**ISBN 978-1-905179-04-6**

**£13.99/$24.99**

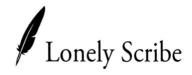
Lonely Scribe

Lightning Source UK Ltd.
Milton Keynes UK
UKOW02f0307290115

245324UK00001B/8/P